Ethical Issues and Patient Rights

Across the Continuum of Care

Joint Commission Mission

The mission of the Joint Commission on Accreditation of Healthcare Organizations is to improve the quality of care provided to the public through the provision of health care accreditation and related services that support performance improvement in health care organizations.

Joint Commission educational programs and publications support, but are separate from, the accreditation activities of the Joint Commission. Attendees at Joint Commission educational programs and purchasers of Joint Commission publications receive no special consideration or treatment in, or confidential information about, the accreditation process.

Contents

Foreword:
page v

Introduction:
Ethical Issues in Health Care
page vii

Chapter One:
Understanding Ethical Perspectives:
A Model for Ethical Inquiry
page 1

Chapter Two:
Application of Ethical Principles and Patient
Rights to Clinical Policies and Procedures
page 19

Chapter Three:
Organization Ethics
page 65

Chapter Four:
Designing and Implementing a Framework for
Clinical and Organization Ethics
page 91

Chapter Five:
Case Study Examples and Discussion Questions
page 119

Resources
page 129

Glossary
page 137

Index
page 147

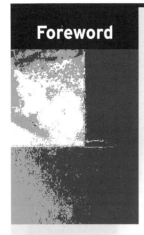

Foreword

Deciding what is ethical behavior—whether for an individual or for an organization—is often not easy. Nowhere is this more true than in health care. After all, health care deals with one of the most personal and important aspects of life——one's own health. It is to be expected that each person has strongly held values about his or her health and about how it should be cared for. At the same time, health care is provided by highly educated and skilled practitioners—doctors, nurses, and others—who have their own sets of values, developed out of the history and mission of their professions. Finally, our society's values include an obligation to provide basic health care for all who are in need.

Because providing health care is such a value-laden endeavor, it is inevitable that different values will come into competition with each other. Health care, therefore, is fertile ground for value conflicts among individuals and groups, and for ethical uncertainty within individuals or groups.

For each of us involved in health care—whether administrator, clinician, or support staff—these value conflicts and uncertainties are a challenge. We *want* to do the "right" thing, but may not know what it is, or how to discover it. And we face these challenges daily in the care of individual patients, in setting policies for the care of patients, and in managing the resources of the organizations in which care is provided. The Joint Commission has recognized these challenges, and the importance of their resolution. For this reason, the Joint Commission has, over the years, established standards that require accredited health care organizations to respect patient rights, to operate in accordance with a code of ethical business behavior, and to make available mechanisms that staff throughout the organization can use to help them resolve ethical conflicts and uncertainties as they arise.

Ethical Issues and Patient Rights Across the Continuum of Care is intended to provide guidance—and examples—of how to recognize value conflicts and uncertainty, how to analyze them, and how to resolve them in an ethical manner. It is designed to assist health care organizations to comply with Joint Commission standards on patient rights and ethics. But this guidance is of use to *all* health care organizations. The public's well-publicized concerns about health care in recent years have often been expressed in ethical terms, resulting in increasing demands not only that every health care organization act ethically, but that they be publicly accountable for their ethical decisions. This book can help health care organizations to address effectively the ethical conflicts and uncertainties they face and to explain the basis for their decisions. We hope this will not only contribute to improving the quality of patient care, but will provide confidence—and comfort—to health care leaders, clinicians and other staff as they resolve the ethical challenges they face.

Paul M Schyve, MD
Senior Vice President
Joint Commission on Accreditation of Healthcare Organizations
Oakbrook Terrace, Illinois

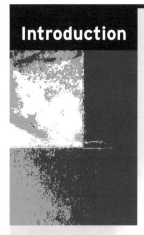

Introduction

In the past 30 years, a number of complex variables have highlighted the need for ethical decision making in the life of most health care organizations. The following list highlights just some of these scientific, political, economic, and social developments:

- Scientific advances in reproductive technology and the care of medically fragile neonates;
- Technological gains in science and medicine that increase life expectancy and prolong life;
- Increased awareness and legal recognition of patient rights, including the right to self-determination;
- A progressive shift in health care financing from fee-for-service to managed care;
- An increasingly diverse cultural, ethnic, and spiritual population;
- A rapidly increasing elder population that is changing the role of members of the nuclear family as caregivers; and
- Changing philosophies toward end-of-life care.

These developments have challenged the prevailing views of the moral obligations of health care organizations and practitioners toward the care of patients. Only a few decades ago, most ethical discussions in health care were limited to the acute care environment, and frequently concerned only questions of self-determination and end-of-life care, dilemmas of treatment alternatives and resource allocation in organ procurement and transplantation, or controversies surrounding clinical research on human subjects.

These concerns certainly remain relevant today as well. However, as health care has shifted from acute hospital care to outpatient services, long term care, home care, and hospice care, the range of ethical questions faced by health care professionals and organizations has exploded. Now the concerns are also likely to focus on business ethics such as resource allocation in a managed care environment, access or admission criteria to certain types of care or reimbursement, and management and staff conflicts of interest. Additional examples of current ethical questions or issues include practice guidelines for palliative care, determinations of decisional capacity for the mentally ill in the community setting or the older adult in a nursing home, appropriate use of reproductive technology, and safe and adequate care of the home health patient.

Basic Questions About Ethics

Although ethical decision making has become an almost-daily challenge across the continuum of health care, many health care professionals express uncertainty and confusion regarding how to approach the process of decision making, and, in some cases, fail to differentiate ethical issues from those that are strictly legal or clinical. The range of questions one might ask in beginning ethical reflection may be multidimensional and are often difficult to answer simply. They may include the following:

- What makes an issue an ethical concern?
- What are the legal and moral obligations, either at an individual or organization level, when responding to a particular case?
- How do we deal with difficult and complex questions of an ethical nature in a more thoughtful manner than simply by giving one's personal opinion or blindly relying on organization policy?
- What relationship, if any, exists between ethical decision making and patient rights? Between ethics and the law? Between ethics and organization risk management?
- Who is responsible for the identification and resolution of ethical concerns as they arise in a health care organization?
- What is the relationship between ethical decision making and good business practice?
- Are ethics committees necessary to solve difficult ethical concerns? What are the organization structures necessary to meet Joint Commission on Accreditation of Healthcare Organizations Rights and Ethics standards?
- What kinds of training do staff need to equip them to respond to ethical decision making thoughtfully and appropriately?
- What will a Joint Commission surveyor look for when evaluating compliance with the Rights and Ethics standards?

The need for ongoing education of health care professionals in the identification and analysis of ethical issues, principles, and values has never been more pressing. Although most health care organizations wish to operate within accepted ethical boundaries, they may not be confident regarding how or where to begin an ethical assessment of their organization. Often the first place to start is by educating staff about basic tenets of ethics and patient rights. Chapter 1 highlights several commonly accepted approaches to ethical theory, including frequently used principles and values such as respect for autonomy, beneficence, nonmaleficence, justice, veracity, fidelity, professional duty, respect for persons, confidentiality, and universality. A case study and a practical framework for ethical analysis using these approaches are also presented.

Patient Rights

As an outgrowth of the civil and consumer rights movements of the 1960s and 1970s, patient rights have similarly gained a heightened prominence in the arena of health care decision making. These rights now include a wide range of considerations, from the right to register a complaint without fear of recrimination or withdrawal of services to confidentiality of medical information to informed consent regarding treatment alternatives. Since the development of patients' rights statements by the Joint Commission and the American Hospital Association in the 1970s, patients and their families have taken an increasingly active role in decisions about their health and the care they receive. In the two decades since the Karen Ann Quinlan case spotlighted the issue of patient self-determination, even when the patient is incapacitated and thus unable to directly make a decision, advocacy groups, professional bodies, and the courts have shaped public policy regarding patient or surrogate participation in end-of-life decision making. The Patient Self-Determination Act of 1990 is a federal law that requires hospitals, long term care facilities, home health agencies, hospices, and other health providers to have written policies and procedures regarding patients' advance directives, including living wills and durable powers of attorney for health care. These health care organizations are further required to inform patients and the community about their right to formulate an advance directive.

Chapter 2 builds on the concept of patient rights and discusses strategies that health care organizations can use to develop internal structures, such as policies and procedures and care processes, to honor them. Sample policies and documents on several of the more complex concerns, such as patient rights, advance care planning, end-of-life care, and determining decisional capacity are included in this section to offer guidance on how a health care organization may want to approach developing or revising similar documents.

Joint Commission Rights and Ethics Standards

The first widely disseminated statement on patient rights was developed by the Joint Commission as a preamble in its hospital accreditation manual in 1971. The statement addressed issues as wide-ranging as equitable and humane treatment regardless of race, color, creed, national origin, or the source of payment for care, patient privacy, confidentiality, and informed consent for technical procedures.[1] By the late 1980s, the Joint Commission began to address patient rights and ethics in its standards, starting with a standard requiring a resuscitation policy in 1988. In 1992, additional standards were added that required the establishment of a mechanism, such as an ethics advisory committee, for the consideration of ethical issues arising in patient care. By 1995, the Joint Commission expanded the patient and resident rights and ethics standards in each of its accreditation manuals, covering topics such as the withholding or withdrawal of life-sustaining treatment, advance directives, informed consent, organ procurement, confidentiality and privacy, the use of chemical and physical restraints, and organization or business ethics.

Organization Ethics

Although ethical decision making in health care has its origins in clinical care, in recent years business and organization ethics have gained recognition as well. Concepts related to organization ethics include establishing organization mission and values statements, conflict of interest policies, codes of professional behavior, and daily operations, all of which model moral leadership and decision making. Chapter 3 offers guidance on issues to consider when designing a framework for organization ethics, including sample values statements and codes of professional behavior.

Ethics Mechanisms

Although ethics committees and consultation services are relatively standard in many hospitals, this type of a formalized ethics mechanism may be new for other organizations across the health care continuum, where the processes for ethics education and decision making tend to be both informal and fragmented. Chapter 4 provides both a sample curriculum for ethics education and a variety of effective educational approaches used in both large and small health care organizations. Considerations for the development, education, role, authority, and evaluation of ethics advisory committees are also presented, and several sample policy and process designs are shared. The Resources on page 129 provide information on a range of educational and consultation resources, from professional societies and ethics centers to books, journals, and reference lists.

Case Study Examples and Guide Questions

The case study approach to ethical analysis has often been one of the most effective teaching strategies, where staff can reflect on both complex and everyday ethics in a pragmatic sense rather than strictly in the abstract. Outside the acute care setting, health care staff frequently think that "ethics" doesn't apply to them because the nature of the issues they confront may not be as "high tech" as care for seriously ill or premature newborns or as complicated as withdrawing a ventilator from a patient in a persistent vegetative state. Yet ethics applies to every setting of health care without exception. Chapter 5 includes a number of hypothetical case studies and guide questions that can be used for staff education and discussion purposes.

The Challenge of Ethics in Health Care

The aim of *Ethical Issues and Patient Rights Across the Continuum of Care* is to help all types of health care organizations face the organization challenges inherent in addressing patient or resident rights and responding to daily clinical and organization ethical questions and demands. This is neither a comprehensive textbook on the theories and principles of bioethics nor an in-depth analysis of individual issues such as reproductive technology or organ transplantation. It is, however, intended to present basic ethical principles and health care values translated into practical strategies for meeting the Rights and Ethics standards of the Joint Commission, including designing educational resources for leaders and staff, ethics committees, policies and procedures, mission and values statements, and patient rights documents.

Now confronted with complex moral questions on a regular basis, health care organizations can no longer afford to view ethics and ethical inquiry as a purely academic or theoretical enterprise engaged in primarily by philosophers. Nor should ethical reflection remain solely the purview of an organization's ethics committee. It is essential that health care leaders, professionals, and staff— which include physicians, nurses, chaplains, social workers, pharmacists, nursing assistants, home health aides, therapists, and dietitians—understand the basic concepts of ethical decision making so that both individual and societal rights and values can be protected and enhanced.

Acknowledgment

We wish to thank all of the organizations who contributed example documents or sample forms; they have shared information which will help other organizations develop or oversee their own ethics mechanisms. We also thank those who devoted time and expertise as reviewers as we developed the manuscript. Finally, our thanks go to Anne Rooney for her outstanding job writing this book. She has presented the complex material in a well researched, understandable, and practical way.

Reference

1. Joint Commission on Accreditation of Healthcare Organizations: *Accreditation Manual for Hospitals.* Chicago: Joint Commission, 1970.

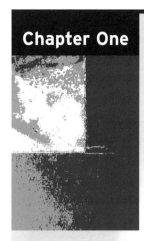

Chapter One

Understanding Ethical Perspectives: A Model for Ethical Inquiry

Health professionals and decision makers are increasingly engaged with ethical problems in a variety of settings, from large teaching hospitals to long term care facilities to smaller community-based hospice programs. Although many health professionals may have at least a passing acquaintance with basic concepts of ethical principles and values, they may feel ill equipped in applying that knowledge to actual patient care or organization situations with any degree of certainty that their conclusions are sound. In some cases, ethical inquiry may serve to raise questions or concerns that are much more complex than the original questions it attempted to address, leaving those involved in the process overwhelmed, confused, or perhaps feeling a bit like they opened the proverbial Pandora's box.

Despite attempts at organizing values, principles, and theories, the discipline of ethics is by its very nature ambiguous. Even well intentioned and caring health professionals may find that often there are no easy answers when "solving" a dilemma, which is of course why a dilemma is a dilemma in the first place. Even if we subscribe to certain organizing principles such as autonomy or beneficence, how are we to know which principle takes precedence, or if in fact one should? How do other values and concerns, such as family or community relationships, religious or spiritual beliefs and practices, life experiences, cultural values, finances, age, gender, home environment, decision-making capacity, organization policies and procedures, and legal considerations enter into ethical reflection? This chapter will discuss those principles and considerations that are frequently used as the foundational building blocks of ethical inquiry in health care organizations, and it will offer a practical model for problem solving and policy development that provides more than simply a consensus of personal opinions around the decision-making table. In Chapters 2 through 4, these concepts will be explored in the context of the standards set forth in the Rights and Ethics chapters of the Joint Commission accreditation manuals.

The Emergence of Bioethics and the Patient Rights Movement

Bioethics, or the application of ethical principles and moral reasoning to the health care arena—including questions raised by medical treatments, advances in health care technology, health care reimbursement, and individual, family, and societal values and beliefs—emerged as a discipline of study in the late 1960s. Its historical roots can be traced to ancient texts such as the Bible, writings of Greek philosophers (Plato and Aristotle) and physicians (Hippocrates), classical philosophers (Immanuel Kant and John Stuart Mill), and ancient and medieval Jewish, Islamic, and Christian theologians. Examples of long-standing theological and ethical beliefs held by most major religions include

- respect for bodily integrity;
- inherent dignity of persons;
- obligations that all human beings share toward one another;
- prohibitions against killing, either another person or oneself;
- doctors' responsibilities to treat their patients; and
- patients' responsibility to seek health care.

The distinction between ordinary and extraordinary means derives from medieval theological thought, when it became established that although an individual must take "ordinary" care of one's life, "extraordinary" measures were not required.[1]

In addition to both philosophical and theological origins, modern ethics and patient rights are also rooted in the liberal political philosophy of John Locke and Thomas Jefferson and seen in such historical documents as the Bill of Rights. This political tradition has been manifested in important legal decisions and regulations, such as the Patient Self-Determination Act of 1990 and decisions based on the principle of privacy, such as the legalization of abortion.[2] According to leading bioethicist-lawyer George Annas, American law is dedicated to fostering individual rights, equality, and justice. It is thus his belief that law, more than philosophy or medicine, is responsible for the agenda and development of American bioethics. Annas contends that the United States, as the most rights-centered society on earth, naturally finds itself defining the issues of personal decision making in terms of constitutional rights; for example, the morality of abortion has been recast as the "right to abortion" and the morality of end-of-life care is now known simply as the "right to die." Furthermore, Annas notes that the case-based common law approach to adjudication of conflicts, namely adjudication by applying principles deduced from previously decided cases to decide current cases, is substantially identical to how many ethical cases are decided.[3]

The concept of informed consent was one of the earliest to emerge in the bioethics literature of the 1960s and 1970s. The concept is based in part on the code of ethics resulting from the Nuremberg trials after World War II, which condemned those physicians who had conducted horrifying experiments on prisoners in Nazi concentration camps. The Nuremberg Code abandoned the older notion that subjects of research should be protected solely by the commitment of the researcher to the subject and replaced it with a notion of self-determination for potential subjects that required informed consent.[4,5] Two subsequent governmental commissions in 1973 and 1983, the National Commission for the Protection of Human Subjects of Biomedical and Behavioral Research and the President's Commission on the Study of Ethical Problems in Medicine and Biomedical and Behavioral Research, provided the first formal governmental analyses of the ethical principles that underlie medical decision making. The mandate of the 1983 President's Commission was a broad one; it dealt with a wide range of issues including care of the dying, genetics, informed consent, and allocation of health care resources.[2] The Commission also published a call to evaluate institutional ethics committees and noted that another type of committee to advise on ethics, the Institutional Review Board, had never received a particularly rigorous assessment regarding its effectiveness.[5]

By the 1970s the bioethics field began to fully emerge with a multitude of issues facing contemporary health care. Among these issues were the legalization of abortion, the landmark Karen Ann Quinlan case that highlighted end-of-life decision-making issues, advances in organ procurement and transplantation, the availability of medical treatments such as cardiopulmonary resuscitation and renal dialysis, and shifts in health care delivery from an acute care medical model to more community-based models and alternative health care approaches. One such alternative model is the development of home-based and volunteer-intensive hospice programs for the terminally ill, which began in the United States in the mid to late 1970s. This emergence was also forged against the backdrop of the civil rights, student protest, consumer, and women's movements of the 1960s and 1970s, in which paternalism or parentalism of all types came under intense public scrutiny. Demands for public accountability and informed consumer decision making represented a profound shift on the political landscape. The "patient rights" health care initiatives of this era were seen by many as an outgrowth of these other political movements. Lastly, the advent of Medicare and Medicaid reimbursement in 1965 radically changed the American health care system—in its payment structure, its laws and regulations, and the physician's relationship to society—and served to heighten the debate about distributive justice and allocation of resources over the next decade.

A new interdisciplinary field of bioethics evolved in response to these questions and developments, drawing individuals from a variety of perspectives, including philosophy, theology, medicine, law, nursing, and medical sociology, among others. Throughout the next two decades, the number and complexity of bioethical issues exploded, ranging from withdrawing or withholding resuscitation or nutrition, to genetic engineering, medical treatments for neonates with congenital anomalies, cost containment and managed care, and fertility and surrogacy debates. Bioethics courses, committees, practitioners, and consultants became a standard component of American health care, law, philosophy, and theology. Patient rights, including informed consent, self-determination through the formulation of advance directives, confidentiality, and the right to complain without threat of reprisal, were widely incorporated into the policies, procedures, and practices of health care institutions. Bioethics today continues not as a single academic discipline, but as a tapestry of rich perspectives, which draws on many sources and bodies of knowledge.

Doing Ethics

Prominent ethicists Thomas Beauchamp and James Childress describe ethics as a "generic term for various ways of understanding and examining the moral life."[6] Hoffman, Boyle, and Levenson define ethics as "systematic and critical reflection on all the steps that make up a moral decision, including assessing the facts, clarifying concepts, and evaluating the force of arguments used to justify a course of action."[7] Ethical theory is often used when referring to thoughtful reflection on the nature of right and wrong. When applied to health care, in which case it is often called *bioethics*, ethics frequently grapples with negotiating a delicate balance between the rights or values of the individual patient, the family or community, health professionals or organizations, and society as a whole.

Reverend Russell Burck, director of the Ethics Consultation Service at Rush-Presbyterian-St Luke's Medical Center in Chicago, describes clinical bioethical inquiry not as just a "debating business" but rather as the "best approximation of the good in this situation." The process of ethical reflection is practical, tests statements about possible alternatives for their ethical acceptability, and provides ethical reasoning to support the conclusion reached. Burck suggests consideration of two fundamental questions in ethical inquiry: What is the "good?" and How do we know? To address these questions, Burck prefers to use the model that Jonsen, Siegler, and Winslade propose in their book *Clinical Ethics*—gathering background details on each specific case, including medical information, the goals of medicine in this case, patient preferences, questions regarding quality of life, contextual matters such as family and staff preferences, institutional policies, and legal standards.[8] In addition, Burck considers the principles that are most important for the case, beginning with respect for autonomy, beneficence, nonmaleficence, and justice. He also includes the need to balance caring versus curing, learn the pertinent narratives of important players, and examine the contribution of virtue and character to the decision-making.

An important perspective on ethics committee work and ethics consultation that Burck considers is suffering, which is often the basis for many requests for case review or consultation. Considering the suffering endured by the patient, family, or clinician during the process of resolving a difficult issue or examining how an issue was resolved can help a committee or consultant explore the issue that is being presented. Often a way to unlock a case is to ask about the pain that the case brings to the person who is bringing the case, or in other words, to ask where the case is "pinching" them.[9]

Daniel Callahan, a pioneering bioethicist and longtime leader at The Hastings Center (Briarcliff Manor, NY), stresses the important role that bioethics should play in examining the "common good" for society as a whole as well as the ethics of one's personal responsibility. For example, what is the individual's responsibility to attempt to stay healthy so as not to burden the taxpayer and society? Because our culture is shaped by the aggregate of individual decisions, it is important to all of us that individual decisions be responsible ones. But who decides what is "responsible"? Above all, Callahan concludes that bioethics should help individuals make good moral choices in their own lives, as in the basic moral question of how ought one to live one's life.[10]

Bioethics is not an exact science, and despite the existence of several widely used decision-making frameworks and principles, there is no single accepted method for "doing ethics." Although bioethics committees and consultation services have contributed greatly to the knowledge and understanding we have about ethical issues in health care, it is far too limiting to define ethical practice by saying, "That's what the ethics committee does." Indeed, most of the ethical life of a health care professional or organization exists outside any established committee format and encompasses the daily practices and values in which patient care is provided. Examples of such daily practices might include respecting the right of a nursing home resident to refuse a certain medication because of unpleasant side effects or evaluating other options and alternatives or in honoring the request of a terminally ill patient to die at home surrounded by loved ones. Examples of values and virtues which are components of ethical behavior include trust, caring, integrity, empathy, compassion, respect, and veracity, or truthfulness.

Educating the Organization

It is essential that education and training efforts, including opportunities to bring forward concerns and conflicts, be extended to all staff of the health care organization. Confining bioethics in a health care organization to the box of an advisory committee structure, which often only makes recommendations on difficult cases or on organization policies, inhibits the rich possibilities in which all staff of the organization can develop and strengthen their own moral compasses. This is not to say that ethics committees do not serve multiple useful purposes. Often one of their key roles, in addition to the more common advisory and policy making, can be to act as a catalyst in fostering an organization climate of ethical awareness, inquiry, and reflection. In addition to their responsibilities with regard to ethical practice and reflection in the realm of patient or resident care, health care organizations as a whole also have an obligation to conduct business ethically as well. Examples of this behavior might be seen in business ventures, billing and reimbursement practices, relationships with payers or the communities they serve, or in the arena of management-employee relations.

Leadership, from governing body members to senior managers and supervisors, plays a key role in creating a climate in which attention to ethics is woven into the fabric and everyday life of the organization. Many health care organizations begin by establishing a values statement that reflects important issues such as trust, integrity, caring, teamwork, accountability, or stewardship. Yet a values statement alone does not create a climate in which organization ethics are understood and honored. It must be a "lived" document, reflecting the manner in which leaders and staff practice in the organization on a daily basis. Organization ethics, including sample codes of ethics, values statements, and conflict-of-interest policies, will be addressed in greater detail in Chapter 3.

In a pluralistic society such as ours, consensus about what is "right" or "wrong" is frequently lacking—especially when it comes to health care. Thus, uncertainties or conflicts around ethical choices inevitably arise, even in the most ethical of organizations or environments. In such situations, a thoughtful analysis of the facts, values, and possible theoretical approaches is useful, both in promoting right conduct on the part of the health care professional or organization and in supporting human fulfillment and dignity. When ethical uncertainties or conflicts exist, it is often because of unclear or competing or conflicting principles, rules, or values. A common conflict is the one between patients' right to make decisions for themselves (autonomy) and the physician's or health care professional's judgment that a particular treatment is not in the patient's best interest (beneficence or the duty to "do good"). Often there are several ethical principles that are central to resolving a complex dilemma of care.

Examining Ethical Issues, Principles, and Values

The following hypothetical case history highlights the story of Mr Brown, a 74-year-old man who is seriously ill with metastatic lung cancer. Mr Brown completed a full course of radiation therapy as well as chemotherapy for treatment of his cancer, and he is now hospitalized with severe shortness of breath and pneumonia. His physician has attempted to manage the symptoms associated with the lung disease, including chest pain, fever, infection, and respiratory distress, but believes that there are no other options available to aggressively treat the underlying cancer. The physician estimates Mr Brown's prognosis to be very poor and his likely survival time to be several months and has discussed this candidly with Mr Brown and his family. Information on advance directives and the availability of palliative care alternatives such as home-based hospice care have been shared with and subsequently rejected by Mr Brown. He recounts his experiences as a prisoner of war during World War II, noting that "I never thought I'd get out of that alive, but God spared me. I think I can beat this thing too. I still have a few miles left in me." Privately, his wife tells his physician that she knows he is dying but that "he's always been a fighter, and it's important for him to still have hope. It would be wrong to take that away from him." Both Mr Brown and his wife clearly state that they "want everything done," including cardiopulmonary resuscitation (CPR), in the event that he suffers a cardiac or respiratory arrest during his hospital stay.

The case of Mr Brown raises a myriad of questions that may appear daunting at first, but with closer analysis we can begin to delve deeper into the issues, principles, and values involved. In other words, it is not hopeless or simply too overwhelming to attempt ethical analysis and resolution in this situation. Among the questions one might ask are the following:

■ As an autonomous individual with the right to self-determination, does Mr Brown also have a "right" to request, even demand, what others might view as medically futile treatment?

■ Does it make any difference from an ethical standpoint if that treatment is one that may potentially prolong his life?

■ How might a physician and other involved health care professionals respond to Mr Brown and his family when they request that CPR be provided, even if the chances of survival to discharge are very slim or if his quality of life will likely deteriorate after resuscitation?

■ What is the physician's moral obligation to Mr Brown, if any?

■ Do physicians also hold the right to autonomy—to practice what they believe is responsible medicine? How does the principle of beneficence impact what physicians do or do not do?

■ Should the rights, values, religious or spiritual beliefs, and life experiences of Mr Brown as an individual *always* supersede the judgments or values of others?

■ How should concerns about distributive justice and wise allocation of resources be factored into the discussion? In other words, who pays, and should that make a difference in deciding the best course of action?

■ CPR is often an expensive treatment option with a documented small survival rate among terminally ill or elderly individuals, and even if the patient does survive the arrest, the result may be an extended stay in the intensive care unit. Does the *potential* benefit to the patient, slim though it may be in terms of medical outcomes, outweigh the burden to society as a whole in such a case?

■ Is it morally necessary to administer medical treatments solely because the patient and family request them?

Taking into account these and other questions, what are the possible approaches to ethics that one might use in problem solving such an ethical conflict?

Ethical theory can provide a framework in which individuals can thoughtfully and systematically reflect on moral conflicts and judgments as well as on the appropriateness of alternative courses of action. Although there is no one universally accepted ethical theory, knowledge and use of one or more acceptable approaches raises the level of discourse above that of mere habit or simple consensus of the personal, and often conflicting, opinions of the decision makers and also adds important insight to the discussion. Such a framework is helpful in building on arguments or principles used in previous cases, as is done in our judicial system of case-based law. A careful ethical analysis provides a greater chance that the conclusions reached will have some measure of internal consistency, even predictability, thus adding to the body of knowledge of bioethics. When considering how an individual, committee, or organization might incorporate ethical theory, it may be helpful to summarize some of the more common approaches currently used in bioethics.

Consequentialism

Also called teleological ethics, consequentialism holds that moral judgments are based on some comparative evaluation of the consequences of possible alternatives and requires that the decision makers weigh the balance of good and bad consequences. It requires that the chosen action be selected based on the alternative that results in the greatest good and the least evil, concepts that, when applied to health care decisions, are often referred to as resulting in the greatest benefit and the least burden. The means used to achieve the outcome are not important in the determination of its morality. Thus, the right act is the one that produces the best overall result, as judged from an impersonal perspective that gives equal weight to all interested parties.[7] *Utilitarianism,* a perspective based solely on the principle of utility or greatest good, is the most prominent of the consequence-based theories and is commonly used in bioethics discussions. Despite its widespread use, consequentialism is not without its limitations and detractors; for example, against what criteria are the "greatest good" determined? What weights will be assigned to the potential burdens or benefits of an action? How will the truly impersonal perspective be obtained?

In the case of Mr Brown just described, a consequentialist might weigh the good and bad effects of administering a medical treatment to a patient for whom it has little chance of success. On the side of the good or benefit, one might want to put Mr Brown's freedom of expression to live out the remainder of his life in a manner consistent with his life philosophy as a "fighter." Hope is important to him, and the knowledge that aggressive medical interventions will be taken to prolong his life will keep that hope alive. Even if the chance of survival from a cardiac arrest is small, it is a matter of a human life at stake, and one argument might propose that the greatest good would be to offer Mr Brown that opportunity for life, no matter how slim. For example, he might want to live to reach some milestone, such as his

50th wedding anniversary, which would provide him and his family with an opportunity to share in an important life event and perhaps resolve past conflicts or estrangements.

Balanced against these potential "good" effects are the "bad" or burdensome ones—for Mr Brown as well as for society as a whole. Considered on an individual basis, CPR could likely have a "bad" effect on Mr Brown's overall well-being because this medical intervention is rarely effective, as judged by survival to hospital discharge of elderly patients who are terminally ill. Mr Brown might die with more pain and suffering from the resuscitation intervention than from the underlying disease. At a societal level, we might consider the resource strain on the health care system that administering CPR would cause. Because Mr Brown is also a Medicare beneficiary, reimbursement for his care will be made from the already-overextended Medicare fund. The net "bad" effect of the burden on society of unnecessary care is that limited health resources are expended in ways that are not likely to promote the health or well-being of an individual or a larger community. It places the individual in opposition to the common good. The aggregate result of many Mr Browns requesting medically futile treatment might be that the Medicare or health care system will eventually be bankrupted, with no resources remaining for public health strategies or preventive health measures.

So what is the "correct" answer to the question of whether or not the greater good is obtained by agreeing to administer CPR to Mr Brown when the consequentialist method is used? As you can see from the range of possible good and bad effects presented, the answer is not a simple one. It is no easy task to try to assign relative weights to each of the possible effects or consequences outlined or to decide in which direction the scale is tipped. Although from a consequentialist perspective, the net "bad" effects, both to Mr Brown and society, would seem to favor *not* performing CPR, this answer still raises questions. We might want to explore still other variables, values, perspectives, and ethical theories before arriving at a recommendation for the hospital, the physician, and the health care professionals caring for Mr Brown.

Nonconsequentialism

This theory of moral judgment is defined by Hoffman, Boyle, and Levenson as one which "holds that there are ways of judging the permissibility of an action, not by a comparison of the consequences, but by adherence to certain values or rules." Moral agents must never commit an evil act or act in an intrinsically evil way so that a good may result. This ethical theory is sometimes equated with a rule-based ethics known as deontological ethics, with the rules or duties emerging from a variety of sources from the Bible to common law or the Hippocratic oath.[7] This approach is also often called Kantian, after the eighteenth century German philosopher Immanuel Kant, whose writings have influenced many of its formulations. Kant saw morality as grounded in reason and rationality rather than conscience or emotion. The moral worth of one's action depends solely on the moral acceptability of the rule or maxim on which the person acts, not on end results of the actions.[6, 11] For example, Kant would find an internal inconsistency, and thus no credit for moral action, in a situation in which a physician lied to a patient to get the patient to agree to a certain course of action that the physician strongly believed was in the patient's best interest because the act of lying is inherently morally wrong, regardless of the good outcome intended by the action.

Kant is also credited with describing moral concepts or values that are now widely accepted in ethical discourse, including universality, autonomy, and respect for persons. Kant's best known rule, described as the *categorical imperative,* proposes that "I must never act except in such a way that I can also will that my maxim (or rule) become universal law." This is sometimes articulated as the concept of *universality.*[12] The example of the physician who lies to a patient to promote a well-intended medical outcome would not pass the test of the categorical imperative because we would never agree that it should be a universal rule that lying is acceptable in some cases, depending on the liar's motives or desirable consequences.

Today we use autonomy to refer to self-governance, self-determination, or even liberty. To Kant, however, people have "autonomy of will" only if they act in accordance with universally valid moral principles that pass the test of the categorical imperative. Autonomy is what gives individuals dignity, respect, and value. Kant's final major formulation is that we must never act to treat any person exclusively as a means to an end, but rather that individuals themselves have inherent worth and thus should be treated with dignity and respect.[6] For example, a victim of a traumatic injury with little chance of survival should never be viewed *exclusively* as a potential donor for organ transplantation, but rather as a person with inherent worth and value whose medical treatment should be decided in his or her best interests, even if the health care providers are also aware of the possibility of procuring precious organs.

Although nonconsequentialism is frequently an implied or commonly held theory in contemporary ethics discussions and problem solving, as with a consequence-based model, there are limitations and complications in trying to determine which rule should take precedence over another in situations in which competing rules or principles may exist. There is no simple formula or cookbook for distilling these competing rules, duties, or principles down to "Rule A always wins over rule B." For example, does truth telling or veracity necessarily carry a greater moral weight than beneficence, which suggests that the physician has a duty to promote the well-being and interests of the patient, in other words, to "do good"? Who decides the relative weights?

If we attempt to apply a rule-based methodology to the case of Mr Brown, the terminally ill patient who is requesting that CPR be administered, we might identify at least some of the rules or duties as respect for personal autonomy, beneficence, nonmaleficence (the duty to refrain from causing unnecessary harm to a patient), justice, and fidelity (the duty to honor commitments or promises). Mr Brown is acting as an autonomous agent, exerting his self-determination through the pursuit of life-prolonging treatments. We might also agree that the physician has a duty of beneficence or, in other words, the promotion of the patient's well-being and interests. A caring and knowledgeable physician might genuinely believe that the administration of CPR to a terminally ill patient does not promote his well-being and might in fact cause more pain, suffering or harm, thus violating the principle of nonmaleficence. In its "Guidelines for the Appropriate Use of Do Not Resuscitate Orders," the American Medical Association (AMA) provides clinical and ethical parameters and strategies to physicians faced with these challenging decisions.[13]

A duty of fidelity may enter our deliberations if the physician and patient agreed at the outset of the therapeutic relationship that the physician would remain as the patient's oncologist until the patient terminated treatment or died. Abandonment of the patient because of a disagreement over treatment options can be seen ethically as a rupture of that verbal contract. The physician is likely to believe that a commitment exists by which he or she should be honest and forthcoming with the patient about the best course of medical treatment. If the physician judges that CPR is not medically appropriate, is there not an imperative that the physician discuss this honestly with the patient? Could avoidance of such an honest discussion then be viewed as a failure to meet the duty of fidelity?

For a number of years, patient autonomy often seemed to serve as the de facto moral "trump card" when decisions of precedence or priority were needed, yet more recent theorists have challenged the advisability of this assumption. For example, Martha Holstein, an expert in bioethics and geriatrics, raises questions regarding even the older patient's preference for autonomy, which is often couched in individualistic terms, when compared to other important values such as community or connectedness. Holstein suggests that traditional notions of autonomy as only an individual issue, rather than in the context of a community such as a family or other residents of a nursing home, may be open to challenges from both research and theoretical analysis.[14] Collopy, Boyle, and Jennings suggest that the dominant orientation of ethics discussions in the acute care setting, namely the protection and respect for autonomous personhood, may not be as easily transferable to the nursing home setting, and recommend consideration of a new approach, that of "autonomy within community." With such a model, autonomy is not seen as strictly individualistic; rather, the person is considered in his or her social context or state of mental capacity.[15] A relatively simple example of this concept in a nursing home might be honoring a resident's personal food preferences when possible, yet expecting this same resident to respect the defined mealtimes of the community. Therefore, the individuals who like to sleep late and eat breakfast at 10:00 AM will need to accommodate their personal autonomy or choices to the needs and rules of the larger community, including mealtimes.

Positivism or Legalism

This ethical theory is described by Hoffman, Boyle, and Levenson as one which "holds that moral norms are in force only if they are adopted or accepted by consent—for example, by a constitution, legislation, or professional codes."[7] Examples of this approach might be acceptance of moral norms in areas such as decision-making capacity or competency, patient self-determination, and privacy as it relates to abortion rights—primarily because of their delineation in law and regulation. One such legal decision that has greatly influenced bioethics in the past decade is the 1990 Supreme Court decision in *Cruzan v Director, Missouri*

Department of Health, which supported a competent patient's right to refuse life-sustaining nutrition or hydration based on the individual's liberty interest.[16] Another example of positivism might be conferring the status of moral norms on certain concepts or principles by demonstrating "substantial compliance" with related Joint Commission standards. In the minds of some organization staff, *compliance* may de facto equate to *ethics,* with limited analysis or discussion.

Although it is certainly beneficial to consider any relevant legal precedents or implications in a particular ethical analysis, the limitations of this approach are that it may not apply to a given situation, the scope of its interpretation may be very small, and it may offer an "easy way out"—the path of least resistance requiring little true reflection. For example, in the hypothetical case of Mr Brown there is no reference in the law to any specific requirement mandating physicians to prescribe medical treatment that they consider futile. A reliance solely on a legal statute in this case would thus provide us with little illumination or direction on how the hospital and physician should proceed.

Another example of positivism is the use of professional codes of ethics, such as those for the medical, legal, social work, dental, nursing, or other professions. Although very useful in setting a general vision and professional ideal, these codes are often not specific enough to be used in analyzing the ethics of an individual case, such as that of Mr Brown. As noted earlier, however, the AMA's guidelines for the use of do-not-resuscitate (DNR) orders might provide useful guidance to the practitioners weighing possible options in this case.

The Ethics of Caring or Feminist Ethics

According to Beauchamp and Childress, an ethics of care "maintains that many human relationships—for example, in health care and research—involve persons who are vulnerable, dependent, ill, and frail, and that the desirable moral response is attached responsiveness to needs, not detached respect for rights."[6] This ethical theory is a relatively new one and is thought by some to be derived from the work of feminist writers studying gender and power in relationships. It focuses on the character traits that are valued in close personal relationships, such as compassion, fidelity, love, friendship, and empathy—concepts that are also discussed in virtue theory. Feminist ethicists often aim for "reasonable opinion" on issues of ethical reflection. As contrasted to consequentialism, utilitarianism, or even Kant's theories of universal moral rules, the ethics of caring has little or no reliance on principles of obligation, rights, rules, or duties. Attachment based on personal relationships, such as that between a family caregiver and the patient, is favored, rather than the detached fairness required in straight ethical analysis. Morality is centered on care and concern, even if this relationship is one between a professional, such as a physician or a chaplain, and the patient and family.[11]

If we attempt to apply the ethics of caring to Mr Brown, we might begin by asking further questions about his family relationships and sense of belonging in his community, religious denomination (if any), and social supports such as the Rotary Club or the Veterans of Foreign Wars. This approach would require that those involved in the ethical reflection get to know Mr Brown and his family to understand his request for CPR in a larger context of relationships, community, and life experiences. For example, perhaps we find out that among Mr Brown's reasons for so adamantly requesting treatment is the expected birth of his first grandchild in seven months or the fact that his wife suffers from a visual impairment and is dependent on him for assistance with activities of daily living. Even though this knowledge will not change the fact than Mr Brown is dying of lung cancer, it will help us to understand his viewpoint in a larger and more textured life context—that of a husband or prospective grandfather rather than simply a hospitalized patient. We might also want to address Mrs Brown's perspective—although she knows that her husband is dying, she believes that it is important that hope not be taken from him and therefore supports his request for CPR. An ethics-of-caring perspective might also question the roles and attitudes of other family members. Perhaps Mr Brown has an adult daughter living across the country who is planning to move in with her parents to help care for her father. What is her view of his CPR request? Active involvement of the patient and family in any discussions using an ethics of care methodology is essential.

Narrative Ethics
In a narrative ethics approach, the patient's or family's story or life narrative is key to understanding the patient's decisions. Each of us exists within a narrative, with a history and a future; medical decisions are part of that narrative. Medical decisions and their consequences can profoundly affect one's sense of identity. In a narrative ethics approach, virtue and character take on particular meaning.[9] Ethicist David McCurdy suggests that attention to the "story" can lead to a deeper respect for patient autonomy and therefore improved care for the patient as a person. Respect for autonomy includes an openness to and appreciation of the values, ideas, and history that lie behind patient choices.[17]

If we apply a narrative ethics approach to the case of Mr Brown, we might identify an event of profound significance in his story or life narrative—for example, his experience as a prisoner of war during World War II. Upon asking further questions about this experience and the impact that it had on him, we might find that he developed a strong sense of personal identity as a fighter and a survivor. This has now become Mr Brown's philosophy of life. In addition to this important fact, we may learn that Mr Brown's son died many years ago from a drowning accident and that immediate medical help was not available to revive him. This piece of his story may influence the way Mr Brown now views aggressive medical intervention. These are just a sampling of the types of information that we might learn about Mr Brown and his life narrative that would influence our further ethical reflection in his case.

A Model for Ethical Inquiry
As one can conclude from this review of various approaches, models, or theories of moral reasoning and ethical decision making, there is no single formula that can be applied to a given situation to automatically determine the right course of action. Ethical reflection is often like detective work in which the decision makers gather as much relevant information about a case or situation as possible and then try to sort through the various conflicts, issues, values, and principles, often

using a hybrid approach of different theories. Sometimes this methodology has even been termed "muddling through," and indeed the process of ethical reflection can at times be frustrating and awkward in the sheer number of issues it raises. Yet each case or discussion can also serve to sharpen our understanding of the complexities of moral decision making, which in the long run is likely to improve both the care and attention patients receive as well as to enhance the ethical climate of the health care organization.

Monsignor Charles Fahey, Executive Director of Fordham University's Third Age Center (Bronx, NY), suggests that before using any particular decision-making process, one should ponder the following questions:

- What precisely is the ethical issue?
- What are the influences at work, and how do they appropriately or inappropriately enter into the decision-making process and affect its outcome?
- Why is a decision necessary?
- What is at stake and for whom? What is the decision's significance?
- Will the decision be temporary or permanent?
- What is the cost, financial or otherwise, of the proposed solution?
- How profoundly will the decision affect the stakeholders' well-being—physical, psychological, and spiritual?
- Who should be involved in the deliberation? With whom should the final decision-making authority reside?[18]

Given the myriad number of facts, principles, and approaches one might confront when analyzing a particularly difficult dilemma, it is often helpful to organize them using a simple model of ethical inquiry. This model might be used by an ethics committee or consultation service, or it might be helpful in a more informal discussion, such as one between health care professionals at a patient or resident case conference or at a hospice interdisciplinary team meeting. The model includes four major components:

1. Gathering and analyzing the facts;

2. Identifying and characterizing the values, principles, or duties involved or in conflict;

3. Exploring the possible choices; and

4. Determining the best possible solution.[19]

Let's summarize each one of these components as we try to draw some conclusions about the case of Mr Brown.

Gathering and Analyzing the Facts

The facts about the case of Mr Brown would include a description of his physical condition, including his cancer diagnosis and treatment history, as well his current pneumonia and physical status, and the goals of his treatment. Other relevant facts about Mr Brown and his family might enter the discussion, such as his decisional capacity, age, military history, spiritual or religious affiliation, and other support systems. An objective reporting of Mr Brown's response to the physician's discussion of advance directives and options for palliative care are relevant here as well. Data or research concerning the survival rates of seriously ill persons who receive CPR, as well as the hospital's policies on withholding resuscitation or on medical futility, might be useful additional information to consider. It is often useful to stress that only the *facts* are what should be considered at this point, so that an individual presenter's interpretation of what they might mean does not prematurely bias the thinking of others. For example, let's assume that in his or her presentation a staff member states, "I bet the reason Mr Brown refused to consider an advance directive is because he thinks that means others would think he is a quitter. My dad is a World War II veteran and he feels the same way." These statements give a personal interpretation of the presenter that does not appear to be based on any objective statement made by Mr Brown. Such an interpretation, whether it is accurate or not, could unfairly bias the thinking of others involved in the discussion and skew the true facts.

Reflecting on the Values, Principles, or Duties Involved

We can summarize the values and principles involved in Mr Brown's case as respect for Mr Brown's personal autonomy or self-determination, the physician's duties of beneficence and nonmaleficence, the principle of distributive justice and wise allocation of health resources, and the duty of fidelity that exists between Mr Brown and his physician. In this step, we might also want to more deeply explore Mr Brown's and his family's spiritual or life philosophy, which is potentially an important value to factor into the analysis. The personal values of the health care professionals, especially Mr Brown's attending physician, are also relevant to consider. For example, Mr Brown's physician may feel strongly that it is unethical to prescribe what he considers medically futile and expensive treatment such as CPR to Mr Brown, because it violates what he believes to be a just allocation of community health care resources.

Exploring the Possible Choices

In our exploration, we may wish to brainstorm as many *possible* choices or alternatives in resolving the conflict or dilemma as possible, even if we agree that not all alternatives are even what we might consider "ethical." Possible choices follow.

■ The physician honors Mr Brown's request for CPR at the present time and orders "full code" on his medical treatment plan.

■ The physician suggests to Mr Brown that a second medical opinion might be beneficial.

■ The physician withdraws from Mr Brown's case because he cannot in good conscience order a medically futile treatment.

■ The physician writes a DNR order in Mr Brown's chart without advising the patient or his family of this order.

■ Mr Brown's caregiving team, including the physician, nurses, social worker, and chaplain hold a patient and family conference to discuss the possible alternatives available to Mr Brown and his family.

Determining the Best Possible Solution

In the case of Mr Brown, it is difficult for us to conclude this step without a thorough analysis and understanding of the three previous ones. At this juncture, it is often helpful to reflect on the various ethical theories or methodologies that might be relevant to the case, so that we avoid having our best possible solution simply be the most expedient or simplistic one, such as "autonomy should always take priority." For example, we might review, as was done earlier in this chapter, how a consequentialist might resolve this case or what conclusions one might draw from a Kantian approach to autonomy and respect for persons. We may end up using a hybrid of approaches, such as blending narrative ethics with a deontological method, and then adding a positivist reference to the AMA's guidelines for the appropriate use of DNR orders.

A broader view of ethical reflection or analysis, using a variety of possible theories, helps to inform our decisions and provides a deeper rationale as to how they were reached. Learning ethics is similar to learning any new skill, whether it be versatility with computers or a new language; it is in working with the concepts, principles, and models on a regular basis that we integrate that knowledge into our daily practice as well as into our own moral philosophies. The consequences of our decision making have profound significance for patients and families, health care professionals and organizations, and society as a whole; therefore, it is imperative that we afford this responsibility the serious reflection, preparation, and practice it deserves. In the next chapter, examples of approaches to patient-related ethical issues are explored in more detail.

References

1. Thomasma DC, Loewy EH: Exploring the role of religion in medical ethics. *Camb Q Healthc Ethics* 5(2):257-268, 1996.

2. Veatch R: Medical ethics: An introduction. In Veatch R (ed.): *Medical Ethics.* Boston: Jones and Bartlett, 1989.

3. Annas G: *Standard of Care: The Law of American Bioethics.* New York: Oxford University Press, 1993.

4. Capron AM, Michel V: Law and bioethics. *Loyola of Los Angeles, Law Review* 27(1):25-40, 1993

5. Wolf SM: Quality assessment of ethics in health care: The accountability revolution. *Am J Law Med* 20(1-2):105-128, 1994.

6. Beauchamp TL, Childress JF: *Principles of Biomedical Ethics,* 4th ed. New York: Oxford University Press, 1994.

7. Hoffman D, Boyle P, Levenson S: *Handbook for Nursing Home Ethics Committees.* Washington, DC: American Association of Homes and Services for the Aging, 1995.

8. Jonsen AR, Siegler M, Winslade WJ: *Clinical Ethics: A Practical Approach to Ethical Decisions in Clinical Medicine,* 4th ed. New York: McGraw Hill, 1997.

9. Personal communication. Rev. Russell Burck, PhD, Director, Ethics Consultation Service, Rush-Presbyterian-St Luke's Medical Center, Chicago, IL.

10. Callahan D: Bioethics: Private choice and common good. *Hastings Cent Rep* 24(3):28-31, 1994.

11. Beauchamp TL, Walters L (eds): *Contemporary Issues in Bioethics,* 4th ed. Belmont, CA: Wadsworth, 1994.

12. Kant I: *Foundations on the Metaphysics of Morals.* New York: Macmillan, 1990.

13. American Medical Association Council on Ethical and Judicial Affairs: Guidelines for the appropriate use of do-not-resuscitate orders. *JAMA* 265(14):1868-1871, Apr 10, 1991.

14. Holstein M: Ethics and aging: A retrospective and prospective view. *Ethical Currents* 48:2-4, 1997.

15. Collopy B, Boyle P, Jennings B: New directions in nursing home ethics. *Hastings Cent Rep* 21(2):1-15 (supp), 1991.

16. *Cruzan* v *Director, Missouri Department of Health,* U.S., 110 S.Ct., 2841 (1990).

17. McCurdy DB: Respecting autonomy by respecting persons: Taking the patient's story seriously. *Humane Medicine* 6(2):107-112, 1990.

18. Fahey C, In American Association of Homes and Services for the Aging Commission on Ethics in Long-Term Care: *Technical Assistance Brief: Attending to the Ethical Dimension of Decision Making.* Washington, DC: American Association of Homes and Services for the Aging, 1995.

19. Rooney AL: Everyday ethics and home care challenges. *Home Health Care Management and Practice* 9(6):31-37, 1997.

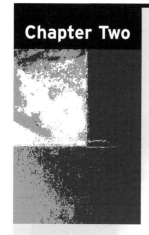

Chapter Two

Application of
Ethical Principles
and Patient Rights
to Clinical Policies
and Procedures

Building on a conceptual and legal foundation of certain core ethical principles, such as respect for individual autonomy, as well as on an assumption that patients or residents have rights deserving of respect, the health care organization must then establish structures to ensure that these are addressed in actual practice. This chapter includes example policies and procedures that demonstrate how ethical principles, legal standards, clinical knowledge, and organization philosophy can be incorporated into developing and implementing policies, documents, guidelines, and processes to meet many of the Rights and Ethics standards in each of the Joint Commission's accreditation manuals.

This chapter is not intended to provide an exhaustive list or representative example of each required policy and process in each Joint Commission accreditation manual. Rather, examples that provide guidance on how policies might be constructed in a variety of health care settings are shared. The examples selected address those areas that tend to be especially complex or subject to change in today's health care environment, especially with respect to the growing public and professional interest in end-of-life care. Of course, any sample policy must be adapted to the needs of the individual health care organization, the patient or resident population served, and specific local or state legal requirements. During an accreditation survey, the surveyors will want to review an organization's policy and will then often interview staff, managers, and patients or residents about how this policy is implemented in practice. For example, the surveyor might review the organization's written patient or resident rights and responsibilities documents and then ask staff to give a practical example of how they honor a particular right, such as the right to privacy or the right to complain without fear of recrimination. During the patient or resident interviews, the surveyor might address the same issue from a slightly different perspective, maybe asking, "How well do you think the organization has addressed your rights with regard to assuring your privacy?" The key to successful integration of the written policies and procedures into actual practice in the organization often lies with ongoing staff and manager education and periodic monitoring, through patient or resident interviews, observations, and feedback, such as the kind obtained through satisfaction surveys.

Table 2-1 (page 22) provides examples of the types of policies, procedures, and documents that a health care organization may want to consider when addressing patient rights and ethics, as well as relevant standards from the Joint Commission's Rights and Ethics chapters. Health care organizations should consider their size, scope of services, and patient population when determining whether the suggested policy, procedure, definition or document meets their needs. Some examples may not fit with the particular scope of services or needs of an organization; for example, a policy on organ procurement would not be appropriate for a home medical equipment supplier, and most long term care facilities would have little need for a policy on the care of seriously ill newborns. The Resources beginning on page 129 present a comprehensive listing of books, journals, ethics centers, training materials, and position statements that are useful in researching and developing organization-specific policies and procedures. Because many of the policies and processes required by Joint Commission

Table 2-1

Checklist for Possible Policies, Procedures, Definitions, and Documents

- ❏ Patient or resident bill of rights and responsibilities
- ❏ Informed consent
- ❏ Participation in investigational studies or research
- ❏ Do-not-resuscitate (DNR) orders
- ❏ Abortion and sterilization
- ❏ Legal guardianship
- ❏ Involuntary commitment and statutory hold
- ❏ Restraint and seclusion
- ❏ Handling roommate conflicts and requests for transfer
- ❏ Criteria for brain death and ensuing practice issues once the criteria have been met
- ❏ Withdrawal or withholding of life-sustaining treatment
- ❏ Medical futility
- ❏ Determining decisional capacity
- ❏ Treatment of seriously ill newborns
- ❏ Confidentiality and release of patient or resident information
- ❏ Handling of complaints or grievances
- ❏ Organ and tissue donation
- ❏ Organ and tissue transplantation
- ❏ Patient HIV (human immunodeficiency virus) antibody testing
- ❏ Refusal of medical treatments, including administration of blood products
- ❏ Special pediatric patient population needs, such as parental cultural or religious objections to recommended medical treatments
- ❏ Advance directives
- ❏ Spiritual needs
- ❏ Palliative care or comfort care guidelines
- ❏ Transfers of patients who are medically stable
- ❏ Handling media inquiries about patients
- ❏ Genetic counseling
- ❏ Assessment and reporting, such as to a protective service agency, of domestic violence, abuse, and neglect
- ❏ Care of patients when staff refuse to participate in care because of religious, philosophical, or cultural reasons
- ❏ Meeting special communication needs of patients

standards, such as for confidentiality and informed consent, are based on both a philosophical and legal premise that patients have certain rights for which they are entitled respect, discussing patient and resident rights is an appropriate first step in policy development.

Rights Documents and Informed Decision Making

Regardless of the setting of care, organization structures must support the rights of individuals or their surrogates to actively participate in decisions about their care, including the right to receive accurate information about their condition and treatment alternatives. The health care organization must also respect and show sensitivity to patient or resident cultural, ethnic, racial, religious, age, gender, language, life-style choices, and needs. The Joint Commission first dealt with ethics in an extensive preamble statement to its hospital accreditation manual in 1971. In 1973, the American Hospital Association (AHA) developed a model Patient's Bill of Rights which has been updated and used as a model for many hospitals since. The most recent revision of this document was approved in 1992 and is included as Figure 2-1 (pages 24 and 25). Health care organizations are encouraged to tailor this sample document to the needs of the community they serve, such as by simplifying the language or translating the document into languages that may be necessary for their patients. The Midwest Bioethics Center (Kansas City, Mo) has also developed a sample patient rights document that includes patient responsibilities for aspects of care, such as the consequences of refusal of treatment or financial responsibilities for hospital charges. This model policy is presented in Figure 2-2 (pages 26 through 28).

The National Association of Home Care has also developed a model patient rights and responsibilities document which addresses areas such as the right to participate in care decisions, the right to formulate an advance directive, the right to confidentiality of medical information, and the right to complain without threat of reprisal or interruption in service.[1] Hospice organizations frequently develop similar documents, adding clauses that address the hospice philosophy for informed consent and truth telling, as well as any organization admission or continuing care requirements regarding the availability of a primary caregiver in the home. The first precept of the National Hospice Organization Code of Ethics provides guidance in formulating patient rights.[2]

Many long term care facilities provide residents with information about their rights in a resident handbook or a commercially printed booklet included in the resident's admission packet. Because the federal and state requirements for addressing resident rights in long term care facilities are too extensive to be reprinted in a sample document here, organizations should consult their state and national professional associations, long term care ombudsman, and legal counsel when drafting their rights document to meet these requirements. The rights document should be comprehensive, addressing such issues as privacy and confidentiality, participation in care planning, transfer and discharge policies, grievances, and the right to and handling of personal possessions, among others.

In addition to distributing rights and responsibilities documents to residents, some long term care facilities may wish to supplement this information with more detailed information addressing areas such as the resident's rights regarding room changes. The Legal Center for People with Disabilities and Older People (Denver, Colo) publishes a number of practical, large-print informational brochures called "Here's Help" on topics such as the inappropriate use of chemical restraints

Figure 2-1	A Patient's Bill of Rights

American Hospital Association

1. The patient has the right to considerate and respectful care.

2. The patient has the right to and is encouraged to obtain from physicians and other direct caregivers relevant, current, and understandable information concerning diagnosis, treatment, and prognosis.

Except in emergencies when the patient lacks decision-making capacity and the need for treatment is urgent, the patient is entitled to the opportunity to discuss and request information related to the specific procedures and/or treatments, the risks involved, the possible length of recuperation, and the medically reasonable alternatives and their accompanying risks and benefits.

Patients have the right to know the identity of physicians, nurses, and others involved in their care, as well as when those involved are students, residents, or other trainees. The patient also has the right to know the immediate and long-term financial implications of treatment choices, insofar as they are known.

3. The patient has the right to make decisions about the plan of care prior to and during the course of treatment and to refuse a recommended treatment or plan of care to the extent permitted by law and hospital policy and to be informed of the medical consequences of this action. In case of such refusal, the patient is entitled to other appropriate care and services that the hospital provides or transfer to another hospital. The hospital should notify patients of any policy that might affect patient choice within the institution.

4. The patient has the right to have an advance directive (such as a living will, health care proxy, or durable power of attorney for health care) concerning treatment or designating a surrogate decision maker with the expectation that the hospital will honor the intent of that directive to the extent permitted by law and hospital policy.

Health care institutions must advise patients of their rights under state law and hospital policy to make informed medical choices, ask if the patient has an advance directive, and include that information in patient records. The patient has the right to timely information about hospital policy that may limit its ability to implement fully a legally valid advance directive.

5. The patient has the right to every consideration of privacy. Case discussion, consultation, examination, and treatment should be conducted so as to protect each patient's privacy.

6. The patient has the right to expect that all communications and records pertaining to his/her care will be treated as confidential by the hospital, except in cases such as suspected abuse and public health hazards when reporting is permitted or required by law. The patient has the right to expect that the hospital will emphasize the confidentiality of this information when it releases it to any other parties entitled to review information in these records.

7. The patient has the right to review the records pertaining to his/her medical care and to have the information explained or interpreted as necessary, except when restricted by law.

8. The patient has the right to expect that, within its capacity and policies, a hospital will make reasonable response to the request of a patient for appropriate and medically indicated care and services. The hospital must provide evaluation, service, and/or referral as indicated by the urgency of the case. When medically appropriate and legally

(continued)

Figure 2-1	A Patient's Bill of Rights
(continued)	American Hospital Association

permissible, or when a patient has so requested, a patient may be transferred to another facility. The institution to which the patient is to be transferred must first have accepted the patient for transfer. The patient must also have the benefit of complete information and explanation concerning the need for, risks, benefits, and alternatives to such a transfer.

9. The patient has the right to ask and be informed of the existence of business relationships among the hospital, educational institutions, other health care providers, or payers that may influence the patient's treatment and care.

10. The patient has the right to consent to or decline to participate in proposed research studies or human experimentation affecting care and treatment or requiring direct patient involvement, and to have those studies fully explained prior to consent. A patient who declines to participate in research or experimentation is entitled to the most effective care that the hospital can otherwise provide.

11. The patient has the right to expect reasonable continuity of care when appropriate and to be informed by physicians and other caregivers of available and realistic patient care options when hospital care is no longer appropriate.

12. The patient has the right to be informed of hospital policies and practices that relate to patient care, treatment, and responsibilities. The patient has the right to be informed of available resources for resolving disputes, grievances, and conflicts, such as ethics commit tees, patient representatives, or other mechanisms available in the institution. The patient has the right to be informed of the hospital's charges for services and available payment methods.

The collaborative nature of health care requires that patients, or their families/surrogates, participate in their care. The effectiveness of care and patient satisfaction with the course of treatment depend, in part, on the patient fulfilling certain responsibilities. Patients are responsible for providing information about past illnesses, hospitalizations, medications, and other matters related to health status. To participate effectively in decision making, patients must be encouraged to take responsibility for requesting additional information or clarification about their health status or treatment when they do no! fully understand information and instructions. Patients are also responsible for ensuring that the health care institution has a copy of their written advance directive if they have one. Patients are responsible for informing their physicians and other caregivers if they anticipate problems in following prescribed treatment.

Patients should also be aware of the hospital's obligation to be reasonably efficient and equitable in providing care to other patients and the community. The hospital's rules and regulations are designed to help the hospital meet this obligation. Patients and their families are responsible for making reasonable accommodations to the needs of the hospital, other patients, medical staff, and hospital employees. Patients are responsible for providing necessary information for insurance claims and for working with the hospital to make payment arrangements, when necessary.

A person's health depends on much more than health care services. Patients are responsible for recognizing the impact of their life-style on their personal health.

This model patient bill of rights was first adopted by the American Hospital Association (AHA) in 1973. This revision was approved by the AHA Board of Trustees on October 21, 1992. It is intended that these rights can be exercised on the patient's behalf by a designated surrogate or proxy decision maker if the patient lacks decision-making capacity, is legally incompetent, or is a minor.

Source: American Hospital Association, Chicago, Illinois. Used with permission.

Figure 2-2	**Sample Patient Rights Policy**
Midwest Bioethics Center	

MD Staff Executive Committee Approval:	Date Effective:
Board of Trustees Approval:	
Chief Executive Officer Approval:	

I. Purpose

The purpose of this policy is to outline the rights of all patients at _____ and their responsibilities. The rights of patients shall also apply to the neonate, child and adolescent patient. The rights of minor patients shall include the parents and/or guardians of these patients.

II. Policy

The patient shall have equitable and humane treatment at all times and under all circumstances. No person shall be denied impartial access to treatment or accommodations available and medically indicated because of disability, race, color, creed, national origin or the nature of the source of payment for his or her care.

A. The patient shall have the right to privacy which shall be protected by the hospital and the attending physician without respect to his or her economic status or the source of payment for his or her care. Individuals not involved in the patient's care should not be permitted access to the patient in any manner which would be detrimental or obstructive to his or her care.

B. The patient's privacy and individual dignity shall be maintained in all areas of examination and treatment within the hospital.

C. The confidentiality of the patient's disclosures, within the law, shall be accorded the patient. This right of confidentiality shall include the right of the patient to decide to participate in the clinical training programs and/or the gathering of data for research purposes. The level of this participation shall not be related to the nature of the source of payment for his or her care except as provided by law or third party payor contracts.

D. The patient has the right to know from those responsible for his or her care:
   1. The identity of the physician who is primarily responsible for his or her care. He or she should know the identity of all individuals participating in his or her care.
   2. The nature and extent of the medical problem.
   3. The planned course of treatment.
   4. The prognosis.
   5. Adequate instruction in self-care in the interim between visits to the hospital or to the physician.
   6. Alternatives for care or medical treatment where medically significant.
   7. Information necessary to give informed consent prior to the start of any procedure and/or treatment and the medical significance of the same.
   8. The probable duration of the hospital stay.
   9. Right to participate in ethical issues that may arise in the provision of his/her care.

E. Communication between the patient and the physician or the hospital should accommodate, where possible, the ethnic, cultural and language variations of the patient.

(continued)

F. In compliance with the Patient Self-Determination Act of 1990:

    1. Adult patients have the right to control the decisions relating to the rendering of their own medical care, including the right to accept or refuse medical or surgical treatment (and to be informed of the possible medical outcomes of his or her action) and have the right to formulate advance health care directives.

    2. No patient shall be discriminated against or have care conditioned on whether or not advance health care directives have been executed.

    3. _____ will comply with state and federal laws governing Advance Directives. Protection of this right shall not be construed to condone or permit any affirmative or deliberate act or omission to end life other than to permit the natural process of dying as defined by statute.

    4. Adult patients have the right to designate a surrogate decision-maker in the event of incapacitation.

G. From the hospital the patient has the right to expect:

    1. A reasonable response to his or her request for services within the capacity of the hospital.

    2. Evaluation, service and/or referral as indicated by the urgency of his or her case.

    3. Complete information and explanation concerning the needs for and the alternatives to his or her transfer to another institution when medically permissible.

    4. Information concerning the relationship of his or her hospital to other health care and educational institutions insofar as his or her care is concerned.

    5. An explanation of his or her bill regardless of the source of payment and to receive information or be advised of the availability of sources of financial assistance, if any.

    6. To be informed concerning hospital rules and regulations applying to his or her conduct as a patient.

    7. Access to his/her medical record information within the limits and specific provisions of applicable law.

    8. Information about the hospital's mechanisms for initiation and resolution of patient complaints or conflicts.

H. No patient shall be discriminated against based on any disabilities as set forth in the Americans with Disabilities Act.

III. Patient Responsibilities

A. *Provision of Information:* A patient has the responsibility to provide, to the best of his knowledge, accurate and complete information about present complaints, past illnesses, hospitalizations, medications, and other matters relating to his health. He/she has the responsibility to report unexpected changes in his/her condition to the responsible practitioner. A patient is responsible for reporting whether he/she clearly comprehends a contemplated course of action and what is expected of him/her.

B. *Compliance Instructions:* Patient Right's Policies often contain a "compliance" clause. These should be reviewed and considered carefully. The following statement taken from the AHA Patient's Rights Guidelines may be helpful.

(continued)

"The collaborative nature of health care requires that patients, or their families/surrogates, participate in their care. The effectiveness of care and patient satisfaction with the course of treatment depend, in part, on the patient fulfilling certain responsibilities. Patients are responsible for providing information about past illnesses, hospitalizations, medications, and other matters related to health status. To participate effectively in decision making, patients must be encouraged to take responsibility for requesting additional information or clarification about their health status or treatment when they do no fully understand information and instructions. Patients are also responsible for ensuring that the health care institution has a copy of their written advance directive if they have one. Patients are responsible for informing their physicians and other care-givers if they anticipate problems in following prescribed treatment."

AHA *Patient's Bill of Rights*, Item 12 ¶2 © 1992 by the American Hospital Association.

C. *Refusal of Treatment:* The patient is responsible for his/her actions if he/she refuses treatment or does not follow the practitioner's instructions.

D. *Hospital Charges:* The patient is responsible for assuring that the financial obligations of his/her health care are fulfilled as promptly as possible.

E. *Hospital Rules and Regulations:* The patient is responsible for following hospital rules and regulations affecting patient care and conduct.

F. *Respect and Consideration:* The patient is responsible for being considerate of the rights of other patients and hospital personnel and for assisting in the control of noise and the number of visitors. The patient is responsible for being respectful of the property of other persons and of the hospital.

IV. Conflict/Complaint Resolution

Patients/families have the right to complain without fear of reprisals about the care/services rendered, and to request that the _____ address these issues.

A. If conflict should occur, the patient/family can request that the physician, nurse manager, chaplain, or social worker serve as the patient/family advocate.

B. If a complaint about service exists, the nurse manager or patient representative will serve as the patient advocate.

C. The patient advocate will be responsible for:
   1. Clearly defining the problem and/or issues.
   2. Bringing together the parties involved in the conflict for the purposes of communication and resolution.
   3. Recommending corrective action to the appropriate authority who will approve, or obtain approval to implement the corrective measures.
   4. Forwarding a copy of the written report describing the conflict to the chairperson of the Quality Improvement Committee of the Medical/Dental Staff, to the Chief Operating Officer of the _____, and to the attending physician.

D. If the concerns or conflict appear related to ethical implications of care, these can be addressed to the Ethics Committee at _____.

This sample patient rights document includes patient responsibilities for aspects of care, such as the consequences of refusal of treatment or financial responsibilities for hospital charges.

Source: Midwest Bioethics Center, Kansas City, Missouri. Used with permission.

in nursing homes, sexuality in nursing homes, and ways of resolving disputes with Medicare health maintenance organizations.[3]

Unique issues often confront behavioral health organizations with respect to client rights and responsibilities. Among these issues are confidentiality of health information (especially between minors and their parents or guardians), restriction or limitation of activities or communications as part of a therapeutic treatment plan, decisional capacity, and the clients' right to refuse aspects of their treatment (such as certain medications). When developing documents and policies in these areas, organizations might wish to research available resources from professional associations, including the codes of professional ethics of organizations such as the American Psychiatric Association, American Psychological Association, and National Association of Social Workers. These codes address issues such as the practitioner's respect for client confidentiality, which might be useful in shaping organization policies and procedures in these areas.

Once the organization determines the patient or resident rights that it will address in the documents or handbook provided to them, it is usually helpful to draft written policies, procedures, and guidelines for those areas that are more complex, have specific legal requirements (such as advance directives or legal guardianship proceedings), or are open to interpretation by staff. The Midwest Bioethics Center's template policy for informed decision making is included as Figure 2-3 (pages 30 and 31). The Center has also drafted an excellent and comprehensive document titled "Health Care Treatment Decision Making Guidelines for Minors," a portion of which is reprinted here as Figure 2-4 (pages 32 through 35). These guidelines can inform health care organizations in thoughtfully drafting policies and rights documents for children, adolescents, and their parents.[4]

Advance Directives and End-of-Life Care

Decision-making at the end of life has been at the heart of many ethical conflicts, discussions, and legal precedents in bioethics in the past 20 years. The landmark legal cases of Karen Ann Quinlan in 1976[5] and Nancy Cruzan in 1990[6] played major roles in highlighting the often complex and difficult choices faced by families, health care professionals, and health care organizations in making decisions about withdrawing life-sustaining care. The Cruzan case especially served as the impetus for the passage of the Patient Self-Determination Act of 1990, which requires certain health care organizations receiving federal Medicare funding (including hospitals, long term care facilities, Medicare-certified home health agencies, and hospices) to provide written information to patients at the time of admission about their right to formulate an advance directive and to provide education to the community about advance directives.

In the early 1990s, a major national research initiative, the Study to Understand Prognoses and Preferences for Outcomes and Risks of Treatment (SUPPORT), spotlighted the ongoing challenges in the care of seriously ill hospitalized adult patients and revealed sobering shortcomings in patient-physician communications around advance care planning and the appropriate use of palliative care. Phase 1 of the study identified significant concerns about patient-physician communications,

Figure 2-3	Template Policy For Informed Decision Making

Midwest Bioethics Center

Medical Executive Committee Approval:	Date Effective:
Board of Trustees Approval:	
Chief Executive Officer Approval:	

I. Purpose

To state the hospital-wide policy on informed decision-making consistent with any legal requirement.

II. Policy Statement

It is the policy of _____ to provide mechanisms that enable the patient to be informed and involved in making decisions about his/her care including:

A. a clear, concise explanation of his/her condition;

B. any proposed treatment(s) or procedure(s);

C. the potential benefit(s) and the potential drawback(s) of the proposed treatment(s) or procedure(s), problems related to recuperation, and the likelihood of success;

D. information should also be provided regarding any significant alternative treatment(s) or procedure(s).

III. Explanation and General Information

A. Information provided to the patient should also include:

    1. Identity of the physician or other practitioner who has primary responsibility for his/her care.

    2. Identity and professional status of individuals responsible for authorizing and performing procedures or treatments, including the existence of any professional relationship among individuals treating him/her as well as the relationship to any other health care or educational institution involved in his/her care. (Cross-reference Patient Rights Policy, Informed Consent Policies as approved by Medical Staff and Board of Trustees.)

B. There should be evidence documented in the medical record that the patient has been given information necessary to enable him/her to make treatment decisions that reflect his/her wishes in accordance with the above Policy Statement, as well as the provisions in III "A". (Cross-reference Patient Rights Policy, Advance Directive Policy, Do Not Resuscitate Policy.)

C. Evidence of informed decision-making for patients undergoing surgical or invasive procedures which require special consent not otherwise covered by the general consent of the patient at the time of admission shall be in accordance with Policy, Use of the Consent to Surgery or Special Diagnostic or Therapeutic Procedure Form, Appropriate Informed Consent Policy, and Action When Appropriate Consent Cannot Be Given By Patient.

D. Discussion of explanation of condition; proposed treatment(s) or procedure(s); the potential benefit(s) and the potential drawback(s) of the proposed treatment(s) or procedure(s); problems related to recuperation and the likelihood of success can

(continued)

Figure 2-3	Template Policy For Informed Decision Making
(continued)	Midwest Bioethics Center

be recorded in the History and Physical, in Progress Notes, consultations, and other portions of the record as appropriate to the timing of the necessary information and decision-making to cover information not addressed by the Surgery/Procedure Consent or other applicable consent forms. It is the responsibility of the physician who performs the treatment/procedure to fully explain proposed plan(s) of care/treatment(s)/ procedure(s) and document patient decision-making in the process.

E. Whenever possible, the explanation to patients should be in "lay" terminology, without abbreviations, and in language or on a level the patient can understand as defined in the Patient Rights Policy.

This template policy details what information should be provided to a patient to ensure that informed decision making regarding care can be practiced.

Source: Midwest Bioethics Center, Kansas City, Missouri. Used with permission.

the frequency of aggressive treatment, and the characteristics of hospital deaths. Only 47% of physicians knew when their patients preferred to avoid cardiopulmonary resuscitation (CPR), 46% of do-not-resuscitate (DNR) orders were written within two days of death, and for 50% of conscious patients who died in the hospital, family members reported moderate to severe pain was experienced by the patient at least half of the time. During phase 2 of the study, a specially trained nurse had multiple contacts with patients, families, and physicians to elicit preferences, improve understanding of outcomes, encourage attention to pain management, and facilitate advance care planning and patient-physician communications. The interventions in phase 2 failed to improve patient outcomes or the care received by patients while they were hospitalized.[7] This study, which was widely discussed and analyzed, served to focus attention on the barriers to the effective use of advance care planning as well as on challenges in the effective care of dying patients. As a result of this new or heightened focus, many hospitals began performance-improvement initiatives focused on these issues. Several examples of such initiatives are shared in this chapter.

In addition, as health care has increasingly shifted from institutional- to community-based care throughout the past two decades, referrals to both hospice and home care organizations specializing in palliative care have increased steadily. In 1983, the hospice Medicare benefit was enacted. It allows patients with a terminal prognosis (a likely survival time of six months or less) to elect to receive hospice care, emphasizing the management of pain and other symptoms as well as psychosocial and spiritual care for the patient and family.[8] Patients who elect the Medicare hospice benefit do so with informed consent and the knowledge that they are, in effect, transferring their payment coverage from their usual Medicare benefits to hospice care. The requirements of the benefit coverage are such that both the patient's physician and the hospice medical director must certify that the patient likely has another six months of life or less, a fact that alone causes many ethical dilemmas for both physicians and for hospice providers. This

Figure 2-4	**Health Care Treatment Decision-Making Guidelines for Minors**

Midwest Bioethics Center

A Patient Rights Statement for Patients With Developing Capacity*

Please read this list of rights. If you need help reading it or need to have some of the words explained to you, ask your mom or dad, someone from your family, or any of the people taking care of you.

This is a list of rights you have as a patient here at _____:

a. The right to be told whatever you need to know to help you understand why you are here.

b. The right to be told in a way you can understand about anything that is going to be done to you while you are here. And to be told truthfully what it may feel like to have those things done.

c. The right to be given answers in ways you can understand to any questions or worries you have about your treatment.

d. The right to tell your family, doctors, nurses and other people taking care of you what you think and feel about your treatment and what is being planned for you.

e. The right to get angry, cry, or say what you don't like about what is happening to you.

f. The right to ask for special things or people who are important to you.

g. The right to know that if you are scared, in pain or hurting, the people taking care of you will always try to help you.

h. The right to help your family and the people taking care of you decide what will be done for you.

i. The right to be given help to solve a disagreement if you and your family or you and the people taking care of you don't agree about what should be done for you.

j. The right to agree or disagree to anything that is going to happen to you. If you tell the people taking care of you that you disagree, to know that nothing will be done to you until the people taking care of you talk to you about our worries and questions.

k. The right to know that nothing will happen to you that you do not want unless your family and the people taking care of you agree that you need to have it done.

l. The right to know that when the people taking care of you touch your body, they will tell you what they need to do, be gentle and do it in a private way.

m. The right to know that what the people taking care of you learn about you will not be told to people who do not need to know.

n. The right to be able to talk freely with the people taking care of you and to know that what you say will not be told to others, including your family, unless it is important to your care.

o. The right to know if your care is part of an experiment. You can agree or not agree to be part of these experiments or stop being part of any experiment.

---

* This statement is written for use primarily with minors who are able to read or to understand its contents if it is read to them. Minors who are infants or pre-school age would not be able to understand the basis of this statement and depend on their family and health care providers to protect their rights. This statement is an inadequate statement of the rights of minors who have decisional capacity.

(continued)

Figure 2-4 | Health Care Treatment Decision-Making Guidelines for Minors
(continued) | **Midwest Bioethics Center**

p. The right to have your family with you as much as possible if you want them to be. When this is not possible, the people taking care of you will explain why they can't be with you.

q. The right to know that nothing done to you by your doctors, nurses or the other people taking care of you is being done to punish you.

r. The right to have the people taking care of you teach you and your family all you need to know about your health care so that you can take care of yourself at home.

s. The right to have a "special safe place."** You will be told about this special place and you and your family will be shown where it is.

t. The right to be treated as a growing person and to have times and places to play and to learn while you are here.

u. The right to read or have this list of rights read to you and explained to you as often as you want.

A Patient Rights Statement for Minors with Decisional Capacity‡

We need you to participate in decisions about your health care. By talking with your care providers and actively participating in planning your care, you will help to ensure that the care you receive reflects your dignity and is in keeping with your desires and values. You are being treated as a person who is capable of making your own health care decisions; therefore, you are being given this information regarding your rights. However, you should be aware that in certain circumstances your ability to act on these rights may be limited by laws, regulations or policies of the hospital. If acting on any of these rights conflicts with the desires of your parents/guardians, you and your parents/guardian will need to work with members of the hospital staff to try to resolve the conflict.

As a patient at _____, you have the right to:

a. Be treated with respect by all personnel.

b. Have your expressed personal, cultural and spiritual values and your beliefs considered when treatment decisions are made.

c. Have a physician primarily responsible for your care and to know who that person is.

d. Know the name and professional status of care givers providing service to you.

e. Receive complete and current information concerning your diagnosis, treatment and prognosis in terms you can understand.

f. Have access to your medical records and to an explanation of all information contained in your records.

g. Have any proposed procedure or treatment explained in terms you can understand. Information you may want includes, but is not limited, to:

** Most organizations which provide care to minor patients provide "safe" areas where diagnostic or treatment procedures are not performed on patients, for example, in classrooms or playrooms.

‡ This statement is written primarily for use with minors who are believed to have capacity to make most health care decisions.

(continued)

Figure 2-4 **Health Care Treatment Decision-Making Guidelines for Minors**
(continued)   **Midwest Bioethics Center**

- a description of the nature and purpose of the procedure or treatment;
- the benefits and risks;
- problems related to recovery;
- the likelihood of success;
- any alternative procedures or treatments (including forgoing specific treatments); and
- costs.

h. Participate with your health care providers in planning your health care treatment.

i. Accept or refuse any procedure, drug or treatment and to be informed of the possible consequences of any such decision.

j. Express your preferences about treatment in advance so that they may be respected should you lose the ability to make treatment decisions. If you choose to write out your wishes, you will be provided information about how to complete advance directives.§

k. Appoint a person to make health care decisions on your behalf in the event you lose the capacity to do so.

l. Have personal privacy. Discussion of your care, consultation, examination and treatment will be conducted discreetly.

m. Have all communications and records related to your care kept as confidential as possible.

n. To be treated fairly regardless of race, color, religious belief, national origin, citizenship, age, gender, sexual orientation, marital status, disability, economic status or source of payment.

o. Receive services in response to reasonable requests that are within the institution's capacity and mission.

p. Be provided supportive care including appropriate management of pain, treatment of uncomfortable symptoms and support of your psychological and spiritual concerns and needs.

q. Receive assistance in obtaining consultation with another physician.

r. Request consultation regarding ethical issues surrounding your care from the institutional ethics committee and other appropriate sources.

s. Be transferred to another facility only after having received complete information and explanation concerning the need for and alternatives to such a transfer. (The facility to which you will be transferred must first accept the transfer.)

t. Consent to or to refuse care that involves research, experimental treatments or educational projects.

u. Complain about our care without fear, or have your complaints reviewed, and, when possible, resolved.

§ In some jurisdictions advance directives made by minors may not be legally binding; however, the task force believes they are important communication documents which should always be considered and honored whenever possible.

(continued)

Figure 2-4	Health Care Treatment Decision-Making Guidelines for Minors
(continued)	Midwest Bioethics Center

v. Be informed by a responsible care provider about continuing health care require-ments and alternatives for meeting those after you are discharged from the health care providing institution.

w. Examine your bill and to receive an explanation of the charges.

x. Be informed of the health care providing organization's policies, procedures, rules and regulations applicable to your care.

If you have questions regarding these rights or wish to voice a concern about a possi-ble violation of your rights, you may contact _____.

_____

This excerpt of patient rights statements for minors can inform health care organizations in drafting policies and rights documents for children, adolescents, and their parents. Written text can be supple-mented by materials more suited for use with children, including children's books and videos.

Source: Midwest Bioethics Center, Kansas City, Missouri. Used with permission.

is particularly true for patients who are seriously and chronically ill with non-cancer diagnoses, such as chronic obstructive pulmonary disease or neurological diseases, in which the prognosis and disease course are often difficult to quantify and predict. Hospices often find themselves faced with difficult decisions regarding access to care and admission criteria, ongoing recertification of the patient's continued appropriateness for hospice care, and (occasionally) patient decisions to revoke hospice benefits to pursue medical treatments that are not considered palliative.

Other common end-of-life ethical dilemmas facing professionals and organizations include the following:

■ Appropriate use of CPR and DNR orders (as discussed in the case of Mr Brown in Chapter 1);

■ Withholding or withdrawal of life-sustaining care or treatment such as ventila-tor support, dialysis, hydration, or nutrition;

■ Truth telling and disclosure of information to patients and families about the patient's diagnosis and prognosis;

■ Refusal of blood and blood products by patients with severe anemia;

■ Appropriate care for dying patients, including comfort or palliative care, with an emphasis on pain and symptom management, psychosocial care, and spiritual care; and

■ Referrals and admission to hospice care.

Advance Care Planning
Since the enactment and implementation of the Patient Self-Determination Act of 1990, which became effective December 31, 1991, health care organizations have searched for successful strategies to

■ provide information to patients about their right to formulate advance direc-tives, such as living wills and durable powers of attorney for health care;

■ offer community education about advance directives; and

■ honor the patient's advance directive once it has ben received.

Fundamental to each of these initiatives has been the conviction that patient autonomy and self-determination should be respected, even if patients are no longer able to make their own health care decisions. The Midwest Bioethics Center developed guidelines and implementation steps to assist health care organizations and ethics committees in meeting the requirements of this federal law. These guidelines are included here as Figure 2-5 (pages 37 through 42). A sample implementation policy, health care treatment directive, and advance directive questionnaire are also included as Figures 2-6 (pages 43 and 44), 2-7 (pages 45 and 46), and 2-8 (page 47). Organizations using these guidelines and sample policy documents will also want to tailor them to any state-specific legal requirements.

Withholding Resuscitation and Other Life-Sustaining Care

As illustrated with the case of Mr Brown in Chapter 1, making decisions regarding the appropriate use of CPR is often a complex process interwoven with multiple variables. Those variables include

■ the physician's best judgments about the usefulness of CPR in individual cases;

■ lack of knowledge about the procedure and its effectiveness by patients and families, often noted in broad statements such as "I/We want everything done" on one side and "I don't want to be hooked up to tubes" on the other;

■ legal and organization policy requirements; and

■ individual and societal values about the use of available medical interventions.

Some ethicists and health care professionals believe that in recent years the focus on patient self-determination and autonomy has resulted in an unfortunate overutilization of CPR in patients for whom it is judged to be medically futile. The emphasis on patient rights may have, in at least some cases, swung the pendulum too far in the direction of supporting patient wishes at any cost, even against best medical judgment. For example, do patients and families have a right to request, even to demand, interventions that are known to be medically futile in some patients? What about the right to request or demand alternative therapies that have no established therapeutic basis? How does one factor in the autonomy of the physician and other health care professionals? Or the common good and societal needs? Should there be a difference in our perspective if the patient is a neonate with multiple anomalies rather than an elderly patient with dementia? Who decides, and based on what criteria?

A number of professional associations, including the American Medical Association (AMA), American Nurses Association (ANA), and American Heart Association, have drafted guidelines or position statements regarding the appropriate use of CPR and DNR orders which are useful references in drafting organization policies and procedures. For acute care or outpatient surgery centers, the policy should also address how a DNR order will be viewed during surgery or

(text continues on page 48)

Figure 2-5	Guidelines for Advance Directive Implementation
	Midwest Bioethics Center

Patient Self-Determination Act of 1990 Guidelines

Implementation Strategies for Ethics Committees in the Development of Policies and Procedures to Comply with U.S. Senate Bill 1766

Purpose

This legislation requires that adult patients be provided with information about their legal rights to make health care decisions, particularly the right to refuse treatment and the right to make advance directives. However, it is clearly the intent of this legislation to encourage health care providing institutions/facilities to enhance patient autonomy and self-determination through a wide variety of steps aimed at education of professionals, patients, and communities.

Definitions

1. *Advance Directive* A general term used in this document to apply to written advance health care treatment directives (sometimes called "living wills") and durable powers of attorney for health care.

2. *Capacity* A person has the functional ability to (1) comprehend information relevant to the particular decision to be made; (2) deliberate regarding the available choices, considering his/her own values and goals; and (3) communicate, verbally or non-verbally, his/her decisions.

3. *Durable Power of Attorney for Health Care Decisions* A signed, dated, and witnessed (or notarized) document which allows an individual to name an agent to make health care decisions in the event the person completing the document becomes incapacitated.

4. *Health Care Treatment Directive* A signed, dated, and witnessed document which allows individuals to state in advance their wishes regarding health care decisions. It is similar to a "living will"; however, it is far more comprehensive than most "living wills." The Health Care Treatment Directive is not necessarily restricted to use only when one is terminally ill.

5. *Living Will* A signed, dated and witnessed declaration by which an individual may request that life sustaining procedures be withheld or withdrawn and that he/she be allowed to die. "Living will statutes" usually apply only when a patient is terminally ill.

6. *Patient Rights* The concept of patient rights can be understood to include a patient's legal rights within a particular jurisdiction; however, a patient's rights also include ethical rights based on duties, obligations and responsibilities of health care providers and institutions. Many health care institutions are required to maintain and to distribute a written "Patients' Rights Statement" which usually includes both legal and ethical rights.

Summary of the Legislation: Under the legislation, Medicare and Medicaid funded providers will:

■ maintain written policies and procedures regarding an individual's rights under state law (whether statutory or recognized by the courts in the state) to make decisions concerning their care, including the right to accept or refuse medical or surgical treatment and the right to formulate advance directives;

(continued)

Figure 2-5	Guidelines for Advance Directive Implementation
(continued)	Midwest Bioethics Center

- ensure that this written information is provided to adult patients at the time of admission as a hospital inpatient or resident of a skilled nursing facility; in advance of coming under care with a home health agency or hospice; or upon enrollment in a health maintenance organization receiving federal funds;
- note in patient records whether an advance directive has been made by the patient;
- ensure compliance with advance directives, consistent with state law;
- provide staff and community education on advance directives.

The Department of Health and Human Services will assist states in developing written information on state law, and will initiate a nationwide public education campaign to increase awareness of advance directives.

Implementation Steps

I. Provide Written Information

A. *To whom?* Information must be provided to all patients age eighteen years or older.

1. Capacity should be assumed and all patients should be provided with information. In situations in which a patient is unconscious, critically ill or otherwise incapacitated, it would be reasonable to provide this information to guardians, family, or other surrogate decision makers and temporarily defer giving information to the patient.

2. It should *not* be assumed that persons who have been adjudicated to be incompetent or diagnosed as mentally ill or mentally retarded are necessarily unable to complete advance directives.

3. Although persons who have permanently lost capacity cannot complete advance directives, information regarding patient rights and relevant hospital policies and procedures (for example, do-not-resuscitate [DNR] policies, and policies and procedures regarding forgoing life-sustaining treatment) should be provided to surrogate decision makers.

4. Legally emancipated minors should be provided with information required under this legislation.

5. This legislation requires that in the case of a hospital this information is to be provided at the time of admission as an "inpatient"; however, hospitals should make reasonable efforts to make this information available to all patients including short-term stay, day surgery, emergency room and other outpatients.

6. Although not specifically covered by the legislation, residents of long-term care facilities admitted prior to December 1, 1991, should be provided this information and the opportunity to complete advance directives.

B. *What is to be provided?* All written information should be available in at least both English and Spanish and written at no higher than an 8th grade reading level. Consideration should be given to making easy to read, large type documents available—particularly in nursing homes.

1. A statement of patient's rights, including
   a. the right to refuse treatment—in accordance with state law
   b. the right to make an advance health care treatment directive (eg, "living will", a health care treatment directive, a durable power of attorney for health, do not resuscitate [DNR] request)

2. A written description of the state law regarding health care decision making.

(continued)

Figure 2-5
(continued)

Guidelines for Advance Directive Implementation

Midwest Bioethics Center

3. Materials developed by the federal government regarding Senate Bill 1766.

4. Written information regarding the institutional/ facility policies regarding implementation of such rights.

5. Information about how to obtain assistance in completing advance directives should also be provided. (Although it is not clear that the law requires providers to assist patients in the completion of advance directives, there is an implied duty to do so.)

C. *When is information to be provided?* Ideally the provision of this information and completion of advance directives should take place when persons are well. One such time might be in the course of a routine visit with a person's primary physician. However, if this has not happened, this process should take place in a setting and at a time when patients can receive information, discuss their concerns, and complete advance directives if they desire. The initial point of contact between the patient and the institution/facility (e.g., the admissions office or the emergency room) is probably not an ideal setting or time for educating patients.

1. *Hospitals and skilled nursing facilities*—the legislation calls for this information to be provided "at the time of admission" which is intended to be defined by institutional policy and may be defined as broadly as to include the admission process.

2. *Home health care agencies*—in advance of individuals coming under care of the agency.

3. *Health maintenance organization*—at the time of enrollment.

4. *Hospice*—at the time of initial receipt of hospice care.

D. *By whom should information be provided?*

1. Information as to whether or not a patient has previously completed an advance directive may be obtained and documented by any member of the staff.

2. Responsibility for providing information to patients as required by this law should be delegated to members of the professional staff who have received appropriate training.

3. More comprehensive education, discussion and assistance in completion of advance directives should also be provided by trained professionals. Social workers, patient representatives and pastoral counselors may play an important role in this process. It is essential for physicians and nurses also to be involved.

II. Elements for Development of Institutional Policies Regarding Advance Directives

A. *Legislatively mandated*

1. Compliance with state laws regarding advance directives

2. Patients' rights statement

3. Non-discrimination provision

   a. Patient may not be denied care as a result of the implementation of an advance directive.

   b. Care of the patient may not be compromised because the patient has enacted an advance directive.

(continued)

Figure 2-5	Guidelines for Advance Directive Implementation
(continued)	Midwest Bioethics Center

4. Conscientious objection clause (Senate Bill 1776—notes that it shall not be construed to negate a conscientious objection clause in any state law).

5. Documentation of compliance with Self-Determination Act should include consideration of the following:

    a. Which member(s) of staff will be responsible for documentation?

    b. Where in the medical record will this information be included?

    c. How will a patient's desire to complete an advance directive be noted and what procedures are needed to respond to such requests?

B. *Important elements not legislatively mandated*

1. It is especially important that the implementation policy include provision for physicians to review all advance directive documents with their patients.

2. Consideration should be given to the relationship between policies for implementing the Patient Self-Determination Act and the institution's/ facility's existing Do Not Resuscitate (DNR) policy, patients' rights statements, and forgoing treatment policies.

3. A procedure should be developed for situations in which the patient or patient's family/surrogate claims that a directive exists but is not produced in a reasonable period of time. A patient with decisional capacity might be asked to complete a new directive.

4. Policies and procedures should include some provision for the resolution of conflicts regarding patient self-determination and the implementation of advance directives. Ethics committees are well suited for this purpose. Guardianship procedures and court determinations should be a matter of last resort.

C. *Incorporation of advance directives into permanent medical records*

1. Mechanisms need to be developed for incorporation of advance directives furnished by patients/surrogates into the patient's permanent medical record.

2. Consideration needs to be given to where in the permanent medical record such documents should be placed, for flagging records which contain advance directives, and for ensuring that copies of advance directives are included in the patient's current chart.

3. Medical record procedures must be developed to allow for the revocation or amending of advance directives maintained in the permanent medical record.

4. Consideration should be given to including information about advance directives in computer data bases.

5. Alternative mechanisms to alert health care professionals to the existence of advance directives (for example, patient identification bracelets, wallet cards and Medic Alert bracelets) could be considered as a means of prompting review of records for such information.

6. Procedures should be developed for transferring advance directive information from patients' charts when a patient is readmitted or transferred to another care unit, institution or facility.

7. Procedures should be developed for providing residents of long term care facilities with the opportunity to periodically review their advance directives.

(continued)

Figure 2-5	Guidelines for Advance Directive Implementation
(continued)	Midwest Bioethics Center

III. Education

A. *Continuing education for staff* Although institutions may choose particular persons or specific departments or services to assume responsibility to act as educators about advance directives, virtually everyone in the institution who patients contact should be prepared to respond to requests for information about advance directives. In addition, it is important that quality assurance, utilization review, risk management and hospital attorneys understand both the letter and the spirit of this significant legislation. Therefore, it is necessary to provide inservice training throughout the institution.

   1. All members of an institution's medical staff should be provided with education regarding both this law and relevant institutional policies developed to implement it.

   2. Consideration should be given to the educational needs of hospital attorneys and risk managers regarding this legislation.

   3. Board members should also be made aware of these important developments in recognition of patient self-determination.

   4. After initial implementation, orientation programs for all new employees and staff should include this information.

   5. Ethics committee members may be appropriate staff educators.

B. *Specific training programs* for professional staff delegated responsibility for educating patients about advance directives should reflect the following:

   1. Education about advance directives is complicated by the psychological difficulty most people have in confronting and working through the possibility of their future incapacity and death. Training for professionals needs to include information and skill development necessary to prepare staff to communicate effectively about these sensitive issues.

      a. Elements of such programs should include effective communication and listening skills, psychological and ethical issues related to death and dying, religious and cultural views, and the like.

      b. Staff training should provide ample time for people to express their concerns and ask questions.

      c. Role playing is an important part of training and should be provided.

   2. Information is made available about the various types of advance directives, i.e., living wills, health care treatment directives and durable powers of attorney.

   3. Information is made available about relevant state law (both statutory and case law).

   4. Information should be provided about the patient Self-Determination Act itself.

   5. Persons trained to educate patients should be knowledgeable about relevant institutional/ facility policies.

C. *Community education recommendations*

   1. Presentations should be short, concise, and made in laymen's terms. The focus of these presentations should be on what advance directives are and what people need to know in order to complete a directive. People should be informed of their rights regarding health care decisions.

(continued)

Figure 2-5	Guidelines for Advance Directive Implementation
(continued)	Midwest Bioethics Center

2. Experts from a variety of perspectives should participate in these workshops and respond to the diverse questions the public may have.

    a. Professionals who may be helpful in these workshops include nurses, physicians, health care attorneys, members of the clergy, patient representatives, social workers and persons trained in clinical ethics.

    b. It may also be helpful to have someone representing administration who can answer questions about the institution's/facility's policies.

3. There should be suitable advance directives provided to people who attend these presentations. (Some institutions have trained personnel available to assist participants to complete advance directives at the workshops.)

4. Relevant policies and procedures should be available. (It will also be helpful to have summaries of relevant state law when they are available.)

5. There should be sufficient time for questions and answers.

6. Community educational programs should provide for special communication needs (e.g., sign language, translators, Spanish speaking, etc.)

D. *Volunteer speakers' bureaus*

1. Ethics centers, the local bar associations and local medical societies often have volunteer speakers' bureaus. Trained speakers may be available, without charge, to churches, civic groups, and other organizations.

2. Institutions/facilities may wish to develop their own speakers' bureaus utilizing ethics committee members or through the training of volunteers.

E. *Educational resources* provided by Midwest Bioethics Center include the following resources:

1. A 17-minute video, *Living Choices,* for use by health care providers and facilities in the implementation of the Patient Self-Determination Act. This film is designed for in-patient education, staff education and/or community education and is already being used nationally.

2. A combined Health Care Treatment Directive/Durable Power of Attorney for Health Care Decisions form.

3. An educational brochure entitled "Making Health Care Decisions for Your Future: Advance Directives" which provides necessary assistance for persons completing the aforementioned document.

4. Inservice training for health care professionals.

5. Speakers for community education programs.

Ethics centers in your area may have other resource materials. For information about this document or any of the services provided, contact Bioethics Development Group, a national division of Midwest Bioethics Center.

The Midwest Bioethics Center developed these guidelines and implementation steps to assist health care organizations and ethics committees in meeting the requirements of federal law for advance directives.

Source: Midwest Bioethics Center, Kansas City, Missouri. Used with permission.

Figure 2-6	Sample Advance Health Care Directives Policy

Midwest Bioethics Center

I. Purpose

Health care providers are required by the Patient Self-Determination Act of 1990 to advise adult patients of their rights to make health care decisions, to formulate advance health care directives, and to accept or refuse medical or surgical treatment. _____ will inform adult patients with capacity about their options and rights to make their own decisions; provide support and assistance to individuals desiring advance directives; and educate patients, professionals and the community. The purposes of this program are to ensure statutory compliance and to enhance patient autonomy and self-determination.

II. Policy

_____ has a systematic, coordinated program to ensure that all adult in-patients with capacity are given the opportunity to develop advance health care directives and that their rights as defined by statutory and case law are protected.

No patient will be discriminated against or have care conditioned upon or compromised solely because an advance directive has been developed.

Advance directive is defined as a "living will," a durable power of attorney for health, a "do not resuscitate" (DNR) request, or a health care treatment directive.

Capacity is defined as the functional ability to (1) comprehend information relevant to the particular decision to be made; (2) deliberate regarding the available choices, considering his/her own values and goals; and (3) communicate verbally or non-verbally his/her decisions.

A. *Goals of the Advance Health Care Directives Program*
1. To inform and educate all adult in-patients about their rights and options under the law.
2. To provide the appropriate documents and to have personnel trained to assist in the execution of the document.
3. To permanently retain documentation in the medical record regarding advance health care directives.
4. To implement the patient's instructions and insure compliance with advance directives consistent with state law.
5. To develop and maintain written policies and procedures regarding individual's rights concerning self-determination and advance directives.

B. *Program Organization and Responsibilities* The overall Advance Health Care Directive Program is under the direction of _____ Administration. Key departments having responsibility for the coordination, management and implementation of Advance Health Care Directives include: Medical Staff, Nursing and Social Work Services.

(continued)

Figure 2-6	**Sample Advance HC Directive Policy**
(continued)	**Midwest Bioethics Center**

III. Procedures

A. *Patient Rights and Responsibilities* All patients admitted to _____ will be provided written Patient's Rights and Responsibilities information and a statement of _____ Law regarding Advance Directives according to administrative policy.

B. *In-Patient Nursing Assessment:*

1. The Admitting Nurse will assess the patient's status and will inquire if the patient has formulated an Advance Directive. If not, the nurse will ask if they wish further information. Response will be documented on the Nursing Admission Assessment Form.

2. If they have an Advance Directive, the nurse will request a copy for the Medical Record. If the document is not currently with the patient, the family/significant other will be asked to bring it to the _____ and route the request for follow up to Social Work Services.

3. If they do not have an Advance Directive but desire further information, the Admitting Nurse will provide the initial packet of information and route the request for follow-up to Social Work Services.

4. If they do not have an Advance Directive and do not wish further information, the Admitting Nurse will inform the patient of their rights to obtain further information at any time.

5. If the patient is unconscious, critically ill, or otherwise incapacitated, documentation will be made of their condition.

6. The Admitting Nurse will complete the Advance Directive Checklist and place it in the Advance Directive section of the Medical Record.

C. *Development of Advance Health Care Directives*

1. The Director of Social Work Services will coordinate an interdisciplinary team of professional staff specifically trained to educate and to assist with advance health care directives.

2. Upon admission referral or specific request, an Advance Directive Team member will be assigned to meet with the patient and provide further education and information to coordinate Advance Directive document activity.

3. If the patient has an Advance Directive which is not available at the time of admission, the assigned staff member will be responsible for attempting to obtain a copy for the current Medical Record. Patients may have an Advance Directive in their physician's office, nursing home or skilled nursing facility, hospice, or home health agency records. These records will be requested from the appropriate file. The patient will be asked to review, revise, reconfirm or revoke the document by signature and date prior to placement in the Medical Record.

This sample policy for advance health care directives meets the requirements of federal law to inform patients of their right to formulate advance directives and to provide support, assistance, and education to patients, professionals, and the community.

Source: Midwest Bioethics Center, Kansas City, Missouri. Used with permission.

Figure 2-7	Sample Health Care Treatment Directive

Midwest Bioethics Center

I, _____, make this Health Care Treatment Directive to exercise my right to determine the course of my health care and to provide clear and convincing proof of my treatment decisions **when I lack the capacity to make or communicate my decisions** and there is no realistic hope that I will regain such capacity.

If my physician believes that a certain life prolonging procedure or other health care treatment may provide me with comfort, relieve pain or lead to a significant recovery, I direct my physician to try the treatment for a reasonable period of time. However, if such treatment proves to be ineffective, I direct treatment be withdrawn even if so doing may shorten my life.

I direct I be given health care treatment to relieve pain or to provide comfort even if such treatment might shorten my life, suppress my appetite or my breathing, or be habit-forming.

I direct all life prolonging procedures be withheld or withdrawn when there is no hope of significant recovery, and I have:

- a terminal condition; or
- a condition, disease or injury without reasonable expectation that I will regain an acceptable quality of life; or
- substantial brain damage or brain disease which cannot be significantly reversed.

1. When any of the above conditions exist, **I DO NOT WANT** the life prolonging procedures which I have initialed below. (You should assume any treatments not initialed may be administered to you.)

   - surgery   _____ initials
   - heart-lung resuscitation (CPR)   _____ initials
   - antibiotics   _____ initials
   - dialysis   _____ initials
   - mechanical ventilator (respirator)   _____ initials
   - tube feedings (food and water delivered
     through a tube in the vein, nose or stomach)   _____ initials
   - other   _____initials

2. I make other instructions as follows: **(You may describe what a minimally acceptable quality of life is for you.)**

   _____

   _____

   _____

If you do not wish to name an agent as referred to on the reverse side, initial here ____, write "None" in the space provided for agent's name, sign and have witnessed and/or notarized.

Discuss this document and your ideas about quality of life with your agent, physician(s), family members, friends and clergy and provide them with a signed copy (or photocopy thereof). *You may revoke or change this document. Periodic review is recommended. If there are no changes after each review, initial and date in the margin.*

(This document is provided as a service by the Kansas City Metropolitan Bar Association and its foundation, the Metropolitan Medical Society of Greater Kansas City, Midwest Bioethics Center and the Missouri Lawyer Trust Account Foundation).

(continued)

Figure 2-7 (continued) — **Sample Health Care Treatment Directive**

Midwest Bioethics Center

Durable Power of Attorney for Health Care Decisions

This is a Durable Power of Attorney for Health Care Decisions, and the authority of my agent shall not terminate if I become incapacitated. I grant to my agent full authority to make decisions for me regarding my health care. In exercising this authority, my agent shall follow my desires as stated in my Health Care Treatment Directive or otherwise known to my agent. My agent's authority to interpret my desires is intended to be as broad as possible and any expenses incurred should be paid by my resources. My agent may not delegate the authority to make decisions. My agent is authorized as follows to:

If there is a statement in paragraphs 1 through 6 below with which you do not agree, draw a line through it and add your initials.

1. Consent, refuse or withdraw consent to any care, treatment, service or procedure, (including artificially supplied nutrition and/or hydration/tube feeding) used to maintain, diagnose or treat a physical or mental condition;
2. Make decisions regarding organ donation, autopsy and the disposition of my body;
3. Make all necessary arrangements for any hospital, psychiatric hospital or psychiatric treatment facility, hospice, nursing home or similar institution; to employ or discharge health care personnel (any person who is licensed, certified or otherwise authorized or permitted by the laws of the state to administer health care) as the agent shall deem necessary for my physical, mental and emotional well being;
4. Request, receive and review any information, verbal or written, regarding my personal affairs or physical or mental health including medical and hospital records and to execute any releases of other documents that may be required in order to obtain such information;
5. Move me into or out of any state for the purpose of complying with my Health Care Treatment Directive or the decisions of my agent;
6. Take any legal action reasonably necessary to do what I have directed.

I appoint the following person to be my agent to make health care decisions for me WHEN AND ONLY WHEN I lack the capacity to make or communicate a choice regarding a particular health care decision and my Health Care Treatment Directive does not adequately cover circumstances. I request that the person serving as my agent be my guardian if one is needed.

If you do not wish to name an agent, write "None" in the space provided below.

Agent's Name: _____ Telephone: _____

Address: _____

If my agent is not available or not willing to make health care decisions for me or, if my agent is my spouse and is legally separated or divorced from me, I appoint the person or persons named below (in the order named if more than one listed) as my agent: **(It is not necessary to name an alternate agent.)**

First Alternate Agent	**Second Alternate Agent**
Name: _____	Name: _____
Address: _____	Address: _____
Telephone: _____	Telephone: _____

Protection of Persons Who Rely on My Agent: I and my estate hold my agent and my caregivers harmless and protect them against any claim for following this durable power of attorney.

Severability: If any part of this document is held to be unenforceable under law, I direct that all of the other provisions of the document shall remain in force and effect.

Signature _____ Date: _____

Witness _____ Date: _____ **Witness** _____ Date: _____

Notarization

Notarization of the Durable Power of Attorney is required in some states (for example, Missouri but not Kansas). If this document is both witnessed and notarized, it is more likely to be honored in other states.

On this _____ day of _____, 199__, before me personally appeared the aforesaid declarant, to me known to be the person described in and who executed the foregoing instrument and acknowledged that he/she executed the same as his/her free act and deed. IN WITNESS WHEREOF, I have hereunto set my hand and affixed my official seal in the County of _____, State of _____, the day and year first above written.

Notary Public _____ My Commission Expires _____

Acceptance (Optional): I have discussed this document with the person making this durable power of attorney and I accept the responsibility designated to me as stated above.

Date: _____ Agent: _____

For more information call Midwest Bioethics Center, 816/756-1735.

This sample health care treatment directive was developed in collaboration between lawyers, clinicians, and ethicists in the Kansas City area. The first page documents decisional capacity and decisions on specific life-prolonging treatments. The second page assigns durable power of attorney for health care decisions for when decisional capacity is lacking.

Source: Midwest Bioethics Center, Kansas City, Missouri. Used with permission.

Figure 2-8	**Advance Directive Policy**
	Provena Mercy Center
Patient Name:	Medical Record #:

Advance Directive Questionnaire

1. **Do you have an Advance Directive prepared?**

Living Will	❏ Yes	❏ No
Power of Attorney for Health Care	❏ Yes	❏ No

If Yes:

Copy obtained from patient/family member	Date: _____
Copy requested from patient/family member	Date: _____
Copy requested from Medical Records (from previous admission)	Date: _____

*Do the patient's wishes as stated on the Advance Directive
represent the patient's current wishes?*   ❏ Yes   ❏ No

*Information to patient/family member: Unless a copy is available for the current chart, the directives cannot be honored unless the patient is able to restate the directive for documentation in the medical record, or formulates a new written directive.

2. **Booklet "Guide to Advance Directives" given to?**

❏ Patient   ❏ Family member   ❏ Other

❏ Unable to give booklet: Reason: _____

Information to patient/family member: If you wish to formulate an Advance Directive, the booklet provides details about the Directives and whom to contact if you wish assistance.

Initials: _____   **Date:** _____

3. **Advance Directive placed on chart at subsequent date:**

❏ Living Will   ❏ Power of Attorney for Health Care

Initials: _____   **Date:** _____

Advance Directive Flowchart

This advance directive questionnaire and accompanying flowchart allow staff to check the status of advance directives for each patient and provide education to patients about their rights to prepare and document an advance directive.

Source: Provena Mercy Center, Aurora, Illinois. Used with permission.

invasive diagnostic procedures. Lifepath Hospice in Tampa, Florida, has developed a policy on withholding or withdrawing life-prolonging procedures (Figure 2-9, pages 49 through 52) which incorporates respect for patient self-determination in end-of-life decisions. It includes specific procedures to be followed in a variety of circumstances, such as when the patient is incapacitated or unable to make a decision and there is no advance directive.

Withholding or withdrawing hydration and nutrition is another common ethical issue faced by hospitals, long term care facilities, home care organizations, and hospices in the care of chronically or seriously ill patients or residents. Professional organizations such as the AMA, ANA, American Society of Parenteral and Enteral Nutrition, and American Dietetic Association, along with others, have developed helpful position statements or guidelines that can be reviewed and referenced in drafting organization policies in this area.

Care of Dying Patients

As noted earlier, the shortcomings in the care of seriously ill patients identified in the national SUPPORT study and the growing public and professional awareness of palliative care and hospice care options at the end of life have focused greater attention on the special needs of dying patients in all health care settings. In identifying the care of this patient population as an unmet or undermet need, professional societies such as the American Geriatrics Society have developed position statements on the care of dying patients. In addition, some health care organizations have selected end-of-life care as a priority for organization performance-improvement efforts, including appropriate pain and symptom management, decisions about withholding or withdrawing life-sustaining treatment, and educating patients, families, and the community about advance directives.[9] The following two examples illustrate such improvement initiatives.

Lutheran General Hospital. In 1996 the Bioethics Committee at Lutheran General Hospital (Park Ridge, Ill) established a subcommittee to explore ways to improve end-of-life care at the hospital, with a particular focus on those patients who were expected to die in the hospital within 72 hours. The subcommittee comprised seven physicians, two chaplains, and one representative each from nursing administration, administration, social work, legal affairs, pharmacy, and clinical ethics. The ethics and pharmacy representatives co-chaired the subcommittee. At its initial meeting, the group identified eight potential areas for improvement and decided to begin by targeting the following three:

1. Guidelines for the development of a palliative care plan;

2. Hospitalwide palliative care policy (Figure 2-10, pages 53 and 54); and

3. Palliative care standing orders.

In one of its improvement efforts, the subcommittee developed palliative care standing orders (Figure 2-11, page 55) to help physicians and other health care professionals take a more comprehensive approach to palliative care and avoid general orders such as "comfort care only." These standing orders are intended to educate physicians and other clinicians as much as to communicate a plan of treatment. The standing orders, by encouraging the physician to consider the

(text continues on page 54)

Figure 2-9	Policy to Withhold and Withdraw Life-Prolonging Procedures

Lifepath Hospice

Subject: Withholding/Withdrawal of Life Prolonging Procedures	Reviewed:	
Department: Program & Services	Effective Date: 5-97	1513
Vice President Approval:	President/CEO Approval:	Revised:

Policy

A. Lifepath Hospice affirms that every competent adult has the fundamental right of self-determination regarding decisions pertaining to his own health, including the right to choose or refuse medical treatment.

B. Any competent adult may make a living will or written declaration directing the providing, withholding, or withdrawal of life-prolonging procedures in the event such person suffers from a terminal condition. Before proceeding with the patient's wishes as designated in the living will, it must be determined that:
  1. The patient does not have a reasonable probability of recovering
  2. The medical condition referred to in the Advance Directive exists
  3. The patient is not pregnant
  4. The patient has a terminal condition

C. Any affirmative or deliberate act or omission to end life other than to permit the natural process of dying is prohibited.

D. *A Refusal of Treatment* must be obtained from the patient, or surrogate or proxy, if applicable, when life prolonging procedures are withdrawn.

E. The patient has the right to revoke a living will at any time, either verbally or in writing. The physician must be informed of this decision.

F. Staff are responsible for providing, or providing for, the education of the patient or legal representative regarding issues of life prolonging procedures. They will respect and support the patient's or legal representative's decisions in these matters.

G. All discussions and education provided to the patient or legal representative must be documented in the Medical Record

H. Staff members who request not to participate in the withdrawal of life support, based on ethical or religious beliefs or cultural values, will be removed from the case if there is no adverse effect to the patient's care or restriction of the patient's right to refuse treatment.
  1. The staff member may not abandon the patient and/or abdicate their responsibilities in the care of the patient until another qualified individual can be assigned.
  2. The Patient Care Manager is responsible for the assignment of back-up staff when the person requesting not to participate in withdrawal is on call.

I. The patient or his legal representative are responsible for communication of their wishes if hospitalized without the knowledge of Hospice. A copy of the appropriate documents should accompany the patient.

(continued)

49

Figure 2-9 **Policy to Withhold and Withdraw Life-Prolonging Procedures**
(continued) **Lifepath Hospice**

Definitions

A. *Life-Prolonging Procedure* Life-prolonging procedure means any medical procedure, treatment or intervention which:

1. Utilizes mechanical or other artificial means to sustain, restore, or supplant a spontaneous vital function .

2. When applied to a patient in a terminal condition, serves only to prolong the process of dying.

3. Does not include the administration of medication or performance of medical procedure, when deemed necessary to provide comfort care or alleviate pain.

B. *Terminal Condition* A terminal condition is a condition caused by injury, disease, or illness from which there is no reasonable probability of recovery and which, without treatment, can be expected to cause death or a persistent vegetative state characterized by permanent and irreversible condition of unconsciousness.

C. *Incapacitated/Incompetent* Incapacitated or incompetent means the patient is physically or mentally unable to communicate a willful and knowing health care decision.

D. *Surrogate* A surrogate is any competent adult expressly designated by the patient to make health care decisions in his behalf upon his incapacity.

E. *Proxy* A proxy is a competent adult who has not been expressly designated to make health care decisions for an incapacitated patient, but is authorized to make health care decisions for him.

Procedure

Withholding of Life-Prolonging Procedures

1. If the physician has ordered a life-prolonging procedure that the patient does not wish to undergo, the patient has the right to refuse.

a. If the patient is incapacitated or incompetent, the surrogate or proxy may decline the intervention, based on the wishes the patient has declared in the living will.

b. If the patient is incapacitated or incompetent, the surrogate or proxy, in the absence of a living will, may make health care decisions for the patient which they believe the patient would have made under the circumstances if capable of making such decisions.

2. The physician must be informed of any decision by the patient, surrogate or proxy, of the refusal to institute life-prolonging procedures.

3. Documentation of the discussion, the decision of the patient, and the notification of the physician must be made in the Medical Record.

Withdrawal of Life-Prolonging Procedures

Competent Patient

A. A request from a patient to withdraw life prolonging procedures must be communicated to the Patient Care Manager and the Risk Manager.

B. The Risk Manager will review the procedure with the patient's primary care nurse (PCN), social worker, chaplain, if any, and the Patient Care Manager.

(continued)

Figure 2-9
(continued)
Policy to Withhold and Withdraw Life-Prolonging Procedures
Lifepath Hospice

C. The Medical Record will be reviewed for the following necessary documents by the Risk Manager and Medical Director:

1. Patient's Living Will.

2. Do Not Resuscitate Order signed by the attending physician.

3. Reports from a physician, hospital history, and physical, pathology or diagnostic testing reports that unequivocally attest to the patient's terminal diagnosis.

4. Written statements from the patient's attending/ treating physician and at least one other consulting physician, who have separately examined the patient. Their findings must support and have determined that:

a. The patient has a terminal condition and may not recover capacity;

b. A medical condition or limitation referred to in an Advance Directive exists.

5. Documentation by the Primary Care Nurse of the patient's request to withdraw life support, the assessment of pain and symptom management, and patient's mental status.

6. Documentation by the Social Worker that the patient is mentally capable, and clearly understands the implications of the decision to withdraw life support. The position of the immediate family must also be documented.

7. *A Refusal of Treatment* form signed by the patient.

Incapacitated/Incompetent Patient with a Living Will

A. A request from a surrogate or proxy** to withdraw life prolonging procedures must be communicated to the Patient Care Manager and the Risk Manager.

B. The Risk Manager will review the procedure with the patient's primary care nurse (PCN), social worker, chaplain, if any, and the Patient Care Manager.

C. The Medical Record will be reviewed for the following necessary documents by the Risk Manager and Medical Director:

1. Patient's Living Will.

2. Do Not Resuscitate Order signed by the attending physician.

3. Reports from a physician, hospital history, and physical, pathology or diagnostic testing reports that unequivocally attest to the patient's terminal diagnosis.

4. Written statements from the patient's attending/ treating physician and at least one other consulting physician, who have separately examined the patient. Their findings must support and have determined that:

a. The patient has a terminal condition and may not recover capacity;

b. A medical condition or limitation referred to in an Advance Directive exists.

5. Documentation by the Primary Care Nurse of the surrogate or proxy request to withdraw life prolonging procedures, and the assessment of the patient's pain and symptom management and mental status.

6. Documentation by the Social Worker that the patient is mentally incapable of decision making, and that the surrogate or proxy clearly understands the implications of the decision to withdraw life prolonging procedures. The position of the immediate family must also be documented.

7. A copy of the Health Care Surrogate's designation.

8. A Refusal of Treatment form signed by the surrogate or proxy.

(continued)

Figure 2-9	Policy to Withhold and Withdraw Life-Prolonging Procedures
(continued)	Lifepath Hospice

D. In the absence of advance directive or designated surrogate, or if the surrogate is no longer available to make decisions, health care decisions can be made for the patient by any of the following individuals (proxy) in the following order of priority, if no individual in a prior class is reasonably available, willing or competent to act:

1. Judicially appointed guardian of the patient, who has been authorized to consent to medical treatment, if such guardian has previously been appointed

2. Patient's spouse

3. An adult child of patient, or a majority of the adult children who are reasonably available for consultation

4. Parent of patient

5. Adult sibling of patient or majority of adult siblings, who are reasonably available for consultation

6. An adult relative of the patient who has exhibited special care and concern for the patient, who has maintained regular contact with the patient, and who is familiar with the patient's activities, health, and religious or moral beliefs

7. A close friend of the patient

E. Any health care decision by the proxy must be based on the proxy's informed consent and on the decision the proxy believes the patient would have made under the circumstances.

1. The proxy must comply with the pertinent provisions applicable to the surrogate

2. The proxy's decision to withhold or withdraw life-prolonging procedures must be supported by clear and convincing evidence that the decision would have been the one the patient would have chosen had the patient been competent.

Conflicts in Care

A. Conflicts between the Interdisciplinary Team (IDT) and the patient's or legal representative's decisions will be referred to the Staff Ethics Committee for review and consultation.

B. If an issue cannot be resolved because of moral or ethical beliefs, the patient will be advised and Hospice will attempt to transfer the patient to another agency within seven (7) days or carry out the wishes of the patient or legal representative, unless in conflict with legislation.

C. If unresolvable conflicts within the patient's family occur, the Interdisciplinary Team will hold a conference with the family in an attempt to resolve the situation. If resolution does not occur, referral will be made to the Staff Ethics Committee for review and consultation.

References: F. S. 765.101-113, 765.201-205, 765.301-310, 765.401; *CAMHC,* Joint Commission on Accreditation of Healthcare Organizations, 1997.

This policy on withholding or withdrawing life-prolonging procedures developed by a hospice organization incorporates respect for patient self-determination in end-of-life decisions. It delineates procedures for competent patients and for incapacitated or incompetent patients with a living will and provides guidelines for conflicts in care.

Source: Lifepath Hospice, Tampa, Florida. Used with permission.

Figure 2-10	Policy on Palliative Care
Lutheran General Hospital	

Subject: Adult Palliative Care	**Effective Date:** 3/1/97
Initiator: Name: 　　　Title:　Director, Clinical Ethics	**Approval:** Name: 　　　Title:　Vice President, Medical Affairs
Supersedes: New Policy	**Review Date:** 19___ 19___ 19___ 　**Approval:** ___ ___ ___

I. Policy

Lutheran General Hospital-Advocate recognizes that in the care of patients with advanced disease it is medically appropriate and ethically acceptable to shift the primary goal of treatment to palliative care if this is judged to be medically appropriate by the patient's physician and consistent with the wishes of the patient or the patient's surrogate.

II. Objectives

The purposes of this policy are to:

A. Clarify the meaning of palliative care, often referred to as "comfort care."

B. Promote comprehensive and consistent palliative care.

C. Establish a process for determining appropriate palliative care for individual patients.

III. Definition

Palliative care consists of all treatments and services aimed at alleviating physical symptoms and addressing the psychological, social, and spiritual needs of patients and their families so as to enhance patients' and families' quality of life to the greatest degree possible.

Palliative care:

■　Affirms life and regards dying as a normal process.

■　Implies the cessation of all diagnostic measures and all life-sustaining and other therapeutic treatments that do not directly contribute to the patient's comfort or to patient and family goals.

■　Consists of active management of pain and other distressing symptoms. In the relief of pain, it is ethically permissible to administer analgesics, in sufficient amounts, to control the patient's pain even if this has the unintended effect of depressing the patient's respiratory function.

■　Is multidisciplinary in order to address the physical, psychosocial, and spiritual needs of patient and family.

IV. PROCEDURE

A. A discussion should be initiated between the attending physician and the patient and/or the patient's family about the appropriateness of shifting goals of treatment to palliative care.

B. The attending physician and other members of the health care team should develop a palliative care plan with the patient and/or the patient's family (usually in the context of a family conference), taking into account their particular goals and needs. Special attention should be given to:

(continued)

Figure 2-10	Policy on Palliative Care
(continued)	Lutheran General Hospital

1. what therapies and procedures should be continued, discontinued or initiated;
2. symptom control, especially the management of pain and anxiety;
3. the most appropriate setting for the patient's death to occur, including the appropriateness of hospice care.

C. The physician should document the patient's and/or family's agreement with the plan in the medical record.

D. The physician should complete the "Palliative Care Order Form." A general order like "comfort care only" is not acceptable.

E. A regular review of the palliative care plan should occur and adjustments made as the patient's condition changes.

V. Endorsements
Medical Staff Executive Committee 11/96
Nursing Executive Team 12/96

After targeting palliative care as a hospitalwide opportunity for improvement, one hospital developed this policy to clarify the meaning of palliative care, promote comprehensive and consistent palliative care, and establish a process for determining appropriate individual palliative care.

Source: Lutheran General Hospital, Park Ridge, Illinois. Used with permission.

---

appropriate discontinuation of more aggressive medical treatments such as parenteral nutrition or dialysis, emphasize that these treatments are now replaced with other interventions and new primary goals of the patient's physical, emotional, and spiritual comfort. The subcommittee continues to meet monthly and is now considering other aspects of end-of-life care, including improving pain management and developing a palliative care team. To assist in evaluating the improvement initiatives it has already undertaken, the subcommittee also uses a medical record review tool (Figure 2-12, pages 56 through 59) to audit the records of terminally ill patients.[10]

Rush North Shore Medical Center. In 1996 the Patient Rights Leadership Team at Rush North Shore Medical Center (Skokie, Ill) presented a list of quality improvement (QI) priorities to the Medical QI Committee. Based on these recommendations, an End of Life Task Force was developed to oversee the improvement efforts of four working teams: the organ and tissue donation team, advance directive team, bereavement team, and DNR–life support team. Membership on the task force and each of the four teams is multidisciplinary and includes representation from across the hospital and medical staff. The task force charged each team with the following responsibilities:

■ Conduct self-education from the literature, standards of practice, and law and regulation;

■ Assess discrepancies between current practice and organization policy;

■ Develop solutions to patient care issues and needs;

(text continues on page 59)

Figure 2-11	Palliative Care Standing Orders

Lutheran General Hospital

(Circle Appropriate Orders)   (Use ballpoint pen only)

DATE HOUR		ORDERS	DATE HOUR	NURSE
	1.	**RESUSCITATION STATUS** This patient is no-CPR. In the event of cardiac or respiratory arrest, cardiopulmonary resuscitation will not be attempted. No "code blue" should be called.		
	2.	**Discontinue all PO and IV medications**		
	3.	**Discontinue IV hydration**		
	4.	**Discontinue all diagnostic procedures and blood draws**		
	5.	**Discontinue ECG and O₂ sat monitoring**		
	6.	**Discontinue supplemental O₂**		
	7.	**Discontinue Parenteral and/or enteral nutrition**		
	8.	**Discontinue arterial lines**		
	9.	**Discontinue central and peripheral venous lines unless required administration of comfort medications as ordered below**		
	10.	**Discontinue PT/OT and respiratory therapy**		
	11.	**Discontinue all blood products**		
	12.	**Discontinue radiation therapy**		
	13.	**Discontinue dialysis (Please notify nephrologist, Dr. _____)**		
	14.	**INITIATE THE FOLLOWING ORDERS TO PROVIDE COMFORT:** **a.** Pain: _____ **f.** Diarrhea: _____ **b.** Anxiety/delirium: _____ **g.** Nausea/Vomiting: _____ **c.** Air hunger/respiratory distress: _____ **h.** Thirst: _____ **d.** Sleep: _____ **i.** Fever: _____ **e.** Constipation: _____ **j.** Other: _____		
	15.	**WITHDRAWAL OF MECHANICAL VENTILATION** **a.** Mechanical ventilation to be withdrawn as follows: _____ _____ **b.** For symptoms of air hunger or anxiety give: Morphine sulfate _____ mg q _____ hr IVP Morphine sulfate 100mg/100ml D5W to infuse at _____ mg/hr Lorazepam _____ mg q _____ hr IVP Other: _____		
	16.	Consult Pastoral Care and Social Work		
	17.	Social Work to evaluate patient for appropriateness of hospice care		
	18.	Transfer Orders:		
		Physician Signature:		

These standing orders for palliative care are intended to educate physicians by encouraging them to consider the appropriate discontinuation of more aggressive medical treatments to meet the primary goals of the patient's physical, emotional, and spiritual comfort.

Source: Lutheran General Hospital, Park Ridge, Illinois. Used with permission.

Figure 2-12	Medical Record Data Sheet
	Lutheran General Hospital

A. Background Information

1. Medical Record Number:_____

2. Date of Birth: _____

3. Gender: ❑ Male ❑ Female

4. Race: ❑ African American ❑ Asian ❑ Latino/Hispanic
❑ Native American Indian ❑ White/Non-Hispanic ❑ Other _____

5. Religion: ❑ Hindu ❑ Jewish ❑ Muslim ❑ Protestant
❑ Roman Catholic ❑ None ❑ Unknown ❑ Other _____

6. Marital Status: ❑ Single ❑ Married ❑ Divorced ❑ Separated ❑ Widowed

7. Date of Admission:_____

8. Date of Death: _____

B. Chart Information

1. Principal Diagnosis:
❑ Congestive Heart Failure ❑ Stroke ❑ Coronary Artery Disease/MI
❑ Sepsis ❑ Renal Failure ❑ Pneumonia
❑ Cancer ❑ Respiratory Failure ❑ Hepatic Failure
❑ Other _____

2. Cause of Death:
❑ Multisystem Organ Failure ❑ Renal Failure ❑ Pneumonia
❑ Heart Failure ❑ Sepsis ❑ Respiratory Failure
❑ Brain Death ❑ Myocardial Infarction ❑ Cancer, specify form _____
❑ Hepatic Failure ❑ Other _____

3. Where did the patient die?
❑ MICU ❑ CICU ❑ Hospital-Hospice Care Unit
❑ GMF ❑ 11 Main-Vent ❑ 8 Center-Cancer
❑ Other _____

4. LOS and on each unit during final admission:
Admitting unit: _____ LOS: _____
Transferred to unit: _____ LOS: _____
Transferred to unit: _____ LOS: _____
Transferred to unit: _____ LOS: _____

C. Advance Directive

1. Did the patient have a living will (LW)?
❑ Yes ❑ No ❑ Unknown/not indicated

2. If yes, was a copy in the chart?
❑ Yes ❑ No

3. Did the patient have a durable power of attorney for health care (DPAHC)?
❑ Yes ❑ No ❑ Unknown/not indicated

If the patient had no written advance healthcare directives (AHCD), skip to section D.

4. If yes to C3, was a copy in the chart?
❑ Yes ❑ No

(continued)

Figure 2-12	**Medical Record Data Sheet**
(continued)	**Lutheran General Hospital**

5. If yes to C4, what treatment choice was specified?
❑ No life sustaining treatments   ❑ Use life sustaining treatments
❑ Use life sustaining treatments,   ❑ None
   except in irreversible coma

6. If yes to C4, were there other specifications on the form?
❑ No   ❑ Yes, what? _____

7. Were the AHCD(s) invoked to make treatment decisions?
❑ Yes   ❑ No   ❑ Unknown/not indicated

8. If yes, how long prior to death were they invoked?
_____ hours/days (circle one)

9. Were the AHCD(s) followed, i.e., were the patient's wishes followed?
❑ Yes   ❑ No, why not?_____
❑ Unknown/not indicated

D. Other Proxy Decision Making

1. Was the health care surrogate act (HCSA) invoked?
❑ Yes   ❑ No

If no, skip to section E.

2. If yes, how long prior to death?
_____ hours/days (circle one)

3. If yes to D1, were the agent's wishes followed?
❑ Yes   ❑ No, why not?_____
❑ Unknown/not indicated

E. Family Conference

A "family conference" is defined here as a discussion between the physician(s) and family member(s) to discuss the goals of medical treatment. The discussion may include additional persons, such as social workers, chaplains, etc.

1. Was there a family conference in this case?
❑ Yes   ❑ No

If no, skip to section F.

2. If yes, how long prior to the patient's death?
_____ hours/days (circle one)

3. Were decisions made to limit treatment?
❑ Yes   ❑ No, why not?_____
❑ Unknown/not indicated

4. What was decided (check all that apply)?
❑ Continue present course of treatment   ❑ DNR   ❑ Comfort care
❑ Everything possible   ❑ Limited time trial   ❑ Unknown/not indicated
❑ Other _____

5. Who was present (check all that apply)?
❑ Patient   ❑ Surrogate   ❑ Family
❑ Guardian   ❑ Physician(s)   ❑ Nurse(s)
❑ Care coordinator   ❑ Social work staff   ❑ Ethics staff
❑ Pastoral care staff   ❑ Other _____

(continued)

Figure 2-12	Medical Record Data Sheet
(continued)	Lutheran General Hospital

F. DNR

1. Was a "no-CPR" order written prior to death?

❏ Yes   ❏ No

If no, skip to section G.

2. If yes, how long prior to death?

_____ hours/days (circle one)

3. When in relation to admission?

❏ Prior to admission   ❏ Upon admission

❏ Post admission, _____ hours/days (circle one)

4. Who was involved in decision (check all that apply)?

❏ Patient   ❏ Surrogate   ❏ Family

❏ Guardian   ❏ Physician(s)   ❏ Nurse(s)

❏ Care coordinator   ❏ Social work staff   ❏ Ethics staff

❏ Pastoral care staff   ❏ Other _____

5. Did the "no-CPR" order impact the use of other medical interventions:

❏ Yes, how? _____

❏ No   ❏ Unknown/not indicated

G. Comfort Care

1. Was there a shift to comfort care?

❏ Yes   ❏ No

If no, skip to section H.

2. If yes, how long prior to death?

_____ hours/days (circle one)

3. Who was involved in the decision?

❏ Patient   ❏ Surrogate   ❏ Family

❏ Guardian   ❏ Physician(s)   ❏ Nurse(s)

❏ Care coordinator   ❏ Social work staff   ❏ Ethics staff

❏ Pastoral care staff   ❏ Other _____

4. What did the physician's order for comfort care say? _____

_____

5. Did the physician's order indicate what treatments should be withdrawn, continued, or initiated?

❏ Yes, specify below   ❏ No

Treatment	Withdrawn	Continued	Initiated
Antibiotics	_____	_____	_____
Artificial Nutrition	_____	_____	_____
Blood Products	_____	_____	_____
CPR	_____	_____	_____
Diagnostic Procedures	_____	_____	_____
Dialysis	_____	_____	_____
Endotracheal Tube	_____	_____	_____
Hemodynamic Support	_____	_____	_____
Hydration	_____	_____	_____
Medications	_____	_____	_____
Oxygen	_____	_____	_____
Pain Relief	_____	_____	_____
Radiation/Chemo	_____	_____	_____
Sedation	_____	_____	_____
Ventilation	_____	_____	_____
Other _____	_____	_____	_____

(continued)

Figure 2-12	Medical Record Data Sheet
(continued)	Lutheran General Hospital

What medications was the patient on at the time of death (list all or check "Unknown"):

❏ Unknown

_____

_____

6. Did the "comfort care" order lead to withdrawal of all medical interventions except pain control?

❏ Yes   ❏ No

7. If no, did the patient continue to receive some treatments generally considered inconsistent with comfort care?

❏ No   ❏ Yes, what? _____

H. Other

1. Did the patient receive curative, aggressive treatment until death?

❏ Yes   ❏ No

2. How many times was CPR attempted on this patient during the final hospitalization?

_____

3. Were pastoral care or social work involved **prior** to death?

❏ Yes   ❏ No   ❏ Unknown/not indicated

4. Was ethics department staff involved in this case?

❏ Yes   ❏ No   ❏ Unknown/not indicated

Other comments:

_____

_____

_____

Data abstracted by: _____   Date: _____

_____

This detailed tool is used to audit the medical records of terminally ill patients. It helps in evaluating the improvement initiatives undertaken by the organization.

Source: Lutheran General Hospital, Park Ridge, Illinois. Used with permission.

■ Develop educational programs for the medical center staff and the community; and

■ Establish baseline data and monitor change.

All of the teams identified significant opportunities to improve both policy and actual practice, as well as to enhance employee, physician, and community knowledge in their respective areas of focus. We will focus on the advance directive team's work here.

The advance directive team began with an educational effort, including conducting a literature review and hosting outside speakers, as well as reviewing the Patient Self-Determination Act, Illinois law and regulations, and local community standards of practice. The team then drafted a flowchart of the process of assessment and communication of an advance directive and identified problems and fail points in the existing process. From that information, the team developed a new flowchart with defined departmental responsibilities and follow-up mechanisms (see Figure 2-13, page 61). Other improvements included

■ development of a new position of advance directive specialist to provide medical center and community education and policy oversight on advance directives;

■ development of a wallet-sized advance directive card for patients to provide information to emergency medical personnel;

■ provision of education to employees, nursing homes, and physician office staff on advance directives;

■ development of a new patient rights and responsibilities brochure (see Figure 2-14, pages 62 through 64);

■ formation of an advance directive resource team within the hospital; and

■ development of an advance directive form in Russian, the primary language for a significant number of the hospital's patients.

Patient-related rights and ethics documents, policies, and procedures are essential building blocks to the foundation of an ethics framework in any health care organization. As addressed in Chapter 4, the organization will need to incorporate education and resources about these polices into staff orientation and ongoing education, as well as into daily patient or resident care processes. In the next chapter, the focus shifts from patient-related ethics issues to those dealing with a broader organization scope, although these issues often affect the care that patients receive either directly or indirectly.

References

1. National Association for Home Care. *Model Patient Bill of Rights.* Washington, DC: National Association for Home Care.

2. The Legal Center for People with Disabilities and Older People. *Here's Help: Your Rights Regarding Transfer, Discharge, and Room Change.* Denver: The Legal Center for People with Disabilities and Older People, 1997.

3. Midwest Bioethics Center: Health care treatment decision-making guidelines for minors. *Bioethics Forum* 11(4):A/1-A/16, 1995.

4. The SUPPORT Principal Investigators: A controlled trial to improve care for seriously ill hospitalized patients. The study to understand prognoses and preferences for outcomes and risks of treatment (SUPPORT). *JAMA* 274(20):1591-1598, Nov 22, 1995.

5. *In re Quinlan,* 70 N.J. 10, 355 A.2d 647 (N.J. 1976) cert. denied, *Garger* v *New Jersey,* 429 U.S. 922 (1976).

6. *Cruzan* v *Director, Missouri Department of Health,* U.S., 110 S.Ct., 2841 (1990).

7. American Geriatrics Society Ethics Committee: The care of dying patients: A position statement from the American Geriatrics Society. *J Am Geriatr Soc* 43(5):577-578, 1995.

8. Public Law 97-248, 122.

Figure 2-13		Advance Directive Flowsheet			
Rush North Shore Medical Center					

Central Registration/ER	YES/Copy available	YES/Copy in previous chart	YES - NO copy available	YES or NO/ Patient from Nursing Home No copy available	NO/Wants more information
1. Does patient have a durable power of attorney for health care or living will?	Copy placed in chart. _____ Date/initials	_____ Date/initials **CALL Health Information Systems x5775** See A	_____ Date/initials **CALL Continuity of Care x5582** See B	_____ Date/initials **CALL Nursing Home Liaison Program x5037** See C	_____ Date/initials **CALL Pastoral Care x5434** NO/Refuses more informa-tion or patient not decisional _____ Date/initials
		(A) Health Information Services Look in old chart for Advance Directive.	**(B) Continuity of Care** Contact family regarding copy of Advance Directive.	**(C) Nursing Home Liaison Program** Call Nursing Home for infor-mation on Advance Directive.	**(D) Pastoral Care** Provide patient information and education on Advance Directive.
		Advance Directive found Copy to Floor/Chart. _____ Date/initials	Copy of Advance Directive released and placed in chart. _____ Date/initials	Faxed copy of Advance Directive placed in chart. _____ Date/initials	Advance Directive completed. Copy in chart. _____ Date/initials
		Advance Directive not found. CALL Continuity of Care x5582 _____ Date/initials	Patient revokes Advance Directive. Document patient revocation. _____ Date/initials	No Advance Directive. Ascertain patient decision capacity. _____ Date/initials	Patient declines Advance Directive. _____ Date/initials
				NO/Wants more information. _____ Date/initials CALL Pastoral Care x5434 NO/Refuses more info or patient not decisional. _____ Date/initials	

This flowchart defines departmental responsibilities and follow-up mechanisms in the process of assessment and communication of an advance directive.

Source: Rush North Shore Medical Center, Skokie, Illinois. Used with permission.

Figure 2-14	Rights and Responsibilities Brochure
	Rush North Shore Medical Center

Patient's Rights and Responsibilities

It is the philosophy of this Medical Center to make our services available to everyone without discrimination on the basis of race, religion, national origin, gender, disabilities or ability to pay.

Patient Rights

1. You have the right to considerate and respectful care.

2. You have the right to obtain from your physician complete current information concerning your diagnosis.

3. You have the right to know the names of your physician and all other persons responsible for procedures, treatment or nursing care.

4. You have the right to refuse treatment to the extent permitted by law and to be informed of the medical consequences of your action.

5. You have the right to privacy concerning your medical care. Case discussions, consultations, examinations and treatment are confidential and will be handled discreetly. Those not directly involved in your care must have your permission to be present during examinations and treatment or during discussions of your case.

6. You have the right to expect that the Medical Center will not disclose the nature or details of your case except to you, to the person making treatment decisions if you are incapable of making those decisions, and to those persons directly involved with providing your treatment. Information may also be disclosed to those individuals processing the payment for your treatment and those responsible for peer review, utilization review and quality assurance. Information will also be given to those parties required to be notified under the "Abused and Neglected Child Reporting Act," the "Illinois Sexually Transmissible Disease Control Act," or where otherwise authorized or required by law. The right to privacy may be waived in writing by you. However, your physician and other health care providers must give you service whether or not you agree to sign such a waiver.

7. You have the right to expect that the Medical Center will make a reasonable response to your request for services. When medically permissible, you may be transferred to another facility only after you have received complete information concerning the need for the transfer. You cannot be transferred to another facility unless that facility has agreed to accept you.

8. You have the right to obtain information concerning the relationship of the Medical center to other health care or educational institutions insofar as such a relationship affects your care.

9. You have the right to know whether research projects that relate to or affect your care are being performed. You have the right to refuse to participate in research projects.

10. You have the right to expect reasonable continuity of care. You have the right to expect to be informed by your physician of continuing health care requirements following your discharge from the Medical Center.

11. You have the right, under Illinois law, to examine and receive a reasonable explanation of your hospital bill, including the itemized charges for specific services.

(continued)

12. You have the right to know that the overriding concern and the very reason for the existence of the Medical Center is to provide the most effective care it is capable of giving.

Advance Directive Information

Durable Power of Attorney for Health Care and Living Will

You have the right to consent to or refuse treatment. Advance directives help assure that your wishes concerning medical treatment are carried out even if you no longer have decisional capacity. Advance directives include the Durable Power of Attorney for Health Care and the Living Will. When you register as an inpatient at the Medical Center you will be given information concerning advance directives.

Durable Power of Attorney for Health Care: This document allows you, while you are still able to make decisions, to designate a person (known as the agent) to make health care decisions on your behalf should you lose your capacity to make your own medical decisions. It also allows you to specify your wishes in advance of illness about what kind of treatment you would prefer in different medical situations, including situations that are not life threatening.

Living Will: This document instructs your physician to withhold or withdraw death-delaying procedures should you develop a terminal condition. If you sign a living will, it will go into effect only when have an incurable, irreversible condition, you are no longer capable of making or communicating health care decisions, and intervention will only serve to prolong the dying process.

You will be admitted to the Medical Center regardless of whether you have an advance directive. The decision to fill out and sign either of these documents belongs solely to you.

Ethical and Patient Concerns

Ethical Concerns

You or your designated decision maker has the right to address ethical concerns that arise regarding specific aspects of your care. These issues may include, but are not limited to conflict resolution, refusal of treatment, withholding resuscitative services and forgoing or withdrawing life sustaining treatment. You or your designated decision maker may request intervention through your nurse, physician, or any staff member. If resolution is not found, you or your family may contact the Director of Pastoral Care. The director will then facilitate an ethics consultation. An ethics consultation can help to focus discussion, open communication, review goals of treatment and identify personal values.

Patient Concerns

All employees of Rush North Shore Medical Center are patient advocates. They are here to ensure that your stay is as pleasant, efficient and effective as possible. Any employee should be able to help your resolve concerns which may arise.

You should feel free to contact the appropriate patient care director, department director or attending physician so they may answer questions and help facilitate a resolution. An administrator is available twenty-four hours a day, and can be contacted through the operator.

(continued)

Figure 2-14	Rights and Responsibilities Brochure
(continued)	Rush North Shore Medical Center

Patient Responsibilities

1. You have the responsibility to provide accurate and complete information about present complaints, past illnesses, hospitalizations, medication and other matters relating to your health. You must report unexpected changes in your condition to your doctor or nurse. You are responsible for making it known if you do not clearly understand your treatment plan or what you must do to aid in your treatment.

2. You are responsible for following the treatment plan recommended by your doctor. This may include following the instructions of nurses and allied health personnel as they carry out a coordinated plan of care and as they enforce applicable Medical Center regulations.

3. You are responsible for promptly fulfilling the financial obligations of your health care. You may be responsible for contacting your employer or insurance company for approval of your stay in the Medical Center or your benefits may be reduced.

4. You and your visitors are responsible for following Medical Center rules and regulations affecting your care and conduct.

5. You are responsible for being considerate of the rights of other patients and Medical Center personnel. You should be respectful of the property of others and of the Medical Center.

References *(continued)*

9. Personal communication. Ron Hamel, PhD, Director, Department of Clinical Ethics, Lutheran General Hospital, Park Ridge, IL.

10. Personal communication. Rev Margaret McClaskey, Director, Pastoral Care and Ethics Consultation, Rush North Shore Medical Center, Skokie, IL.

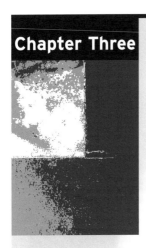

Chapter Three

Organization
Ethics

Much of the discussion concerning ethical decision making in health care organizations in the past 30 years has concerned the values, principles, conflicts, and dilemmas surrounding the care of the patient—often with a special emphasis on the practitioner's or clinician's professional responsibility to the patient. Principles and values such as patient autonomy or the professional's responsibility to enact beneficence or to "do good" frequently have served as the cornerstones for ethical reflection within the organization. Even if the conflict or dilemma involved the organization's ethical responsibilities rather than those of a single clinician, these usually were framed in the context of a particular patient situation or set of clinical circumstances such as end-of-life decision making.

Integrating Clinical and Organization Ethics
In recent years the topic of organization ethics has come into its own as a unique set of challenges, largely because of sweeping societal changes in the health care delivery system. Prominent among these changes are the explosion of managed care, the increasing vertical integration of health care organizations, partnerships between health care organizations and physicians, health care marketing and strategic planning initiatives, and mergers and acquisitions of both small and large health care organizations. Business ethics and codes of ethical conduct in all types of organizations have gained public interest and scrutiny in the past decade, ranging from the ethical behavior of elected officials to the integrity of a Wall Street securities firm. Expanding government activities that target potential fraud and abuse in health care reimbursement and billing practices have focused national attention on the business practices and ethics of health care organizations.

Never before in their history have health care organizations faced such profound external pressures on their survival, pressures which at times place the mission of the organization to serve the community in direct conflict with its financial viability. The health care organization may have a mission to provide care to those who need it regardless of ability to pay, yet without some source of financial support, usually third-party reimbursement, the organization cannot continue to offer both the service to the patient as well as ongoing employment to its workers. An ethical conflict often develops as a result of the dueling choices of patient care needs and the organization's financial solvency. This dilemma is especially significant in many of our large urban and public health care institutions. Can an ethical organization culture coexist with meeting the external demands of the health care reimbursement system? With moral leadership and a deep commitment to integrating core values into daily operations, such a culture can not only exist but also thrive.

Nurturing an Ethical Climate Within a Health Care Organization
An ethical organization culture cannot be created through mere policy statements, buzzwords, or slogans such as Do the Right Thing. An ethical culture is an outgrowth of processes, policies, and leadership that support and integrate key values such as fairness, integrity, and trust into the daily life of the organization. An ethical culture is developed cumulatively, building on lived experiences, behaviors,

and interpersonal interactions. Conversely, obvious disparity between what is espoused in a written values statement and what employees experience in practice will detour the organization's ethical journey and lead to cynicism and mistrust. Building an ethical climate requires nurturance and thoughtful reflection.

In short, there is no quick recipe or formula for creation of an ethical climate. An ethical framework is not a document, but rather a way of relating with others both within and outside the organization—the way an organization does business and conducts its activities in all aspects of organization life. In the process of the evolution of a new organization climate, it is often helpful to periodically monitor the progress toward achieving the goal of an ethical climate. Leaders may find the following questions useful guideposts for assessing and enhancing the ethical climate of the organization.

■ Does the organization have a written mission and values or ethics statement that has been shared with all staff, including physicians? Is this statement available to the public as well, so that the community can help to monitor its implementation in practice?

■ Does the values statement or its interpretation provide practical illustrations and advice on how the core values can be integrated into daily practice?

■ Is there alignment between the organization's values and its written policies and procedures in areas such as administration, patient care, human resource management, marketing, and billing? Between the values and contractual relationships or partnerships with other organizations or individuals?

■ By what behaviors do the leaders serve as role models of the organization's core values? Are there disparities between what is supported verbally or conceptually and what is practiced in daily operations?

■ Does the organization have a conflict-of-interest statement for all leaders and staff? Is it understood and supported? By what mechanism are conflicts disclosed and addressed?

■ How is exemplary ethical conduct rewarded in the organization?

■ How are ethical violations or misconduct addressed? Does the organization have controls in place to monitor for these violations?

■ Are ethical values addressed in human resource management practices, such as promotions or performance appraisals?

■ What ongoing mechanisms for supporting an ethical organization climate, such as open ethics forums, staff education and training programs, and employee handbooks are in place? How are new ethical challenges identified?

Some health care organizations have designed innovative values-centered or ethical leadership training for all senior and middle managers as a method of integrating ethical principles into daily management decision making. Yet in many cases, the paradigm shift from considering ethics in a strictly clinical context to a broader organization realm, including human resource management, information management, and financial management, might not come easily. Clinical ethicist Robert Lyman Potter notes that the typical ethics committee is not prepared for, and may even be resistant to, the task of organization ethics, because the committee's role is often focused narrowly on clinical case consultation with a relative neglect of education and policy development. Potter proposes that health care organizations consider an integrated ethics mechanism that includes at its core an augmented ethics committee positioned to introduce ethical decision making at every level throughout the organization. He defines such a program as one that is an "integration of clinical and corporate ethics which engages all levels and functions of the organization into one value vision of making ethics as important for health care decisions as clinical data, financial concerns, and legal issues."[1]

Some health care organizations with well-established ethics mechanisms such as a committee or ethics forum have found it both possible and effective to expand the role of the committee from one of primarily case consultation to one that proactively involves both clinical and administrative policy development on ethical concerns and principles. Paul Schyve, senior vice president of the Joint Commission, suggests that effective members of ethics committees have skills which are often transferable to the realm of organization and business ethics, including knowledge of ethical principles and how to reason about ethical questions, skills in communicating and educating about these principles, and skills in facilitating ethical dialogue and decision making.[2]

In expanding the role of an existing ethics committee that functions in a clinical consultation or advisory capacity, it is usually necessary to provide additional training and resources to committee members to prepare them for this responsibility. In larger or more complex health care organizations, such as tertiary care centers, maintaining two distinct functions—clinical ethics and organization ethics—might be the most effective approach, owing to the often-complicated nature of the issues that these organizations face. In such situations, a liaison between these two functions is needed because decisions in one area will likely have implications for the other. In smaller organizations, such as a long term care facility or a home health agency, identification and analysis of organization ethical concerns is often done informally by the management team, with input from staff through surveys or staff meetings.

Whatever methods or structures are selected, it is essential that staff and employees not see "organization ethics" as mere words on a values statement, the latest in customer-focused marketing techniques, or empty codes that are not upheld in the daily life of the organization. Just as with the concept of quality improvement, leaders in the organization must first model the ethical behavior they expect to be followed by others. However, although the leaders' commitment to ethical behavior is essential, no one is exempted from ethical responsibility, whether or not leaders or peers are acting ethically. Practicing ethical behavior is both an individual and organization imperative.

In 1991, the Woodstock Theological Center, a nonprofit research institute in Washington, DC, convened a diverse group of national health care leaders, including executives, physicians, nurses, ethicists, religious leaders, and academicians, to address issues of social or political importance from an ethical perspective and to formulate a consensus statement on ethical considerations in the business aspects of health care. Meeting several times throughout the next two years, the seminar group identified, grouped, and analyzed the most common ethical issues confronting health care professionals related to the business aspect of health care and developed a set of principles for use in addressing them. The core principles formulated by the seminar participants follow.

- *Compassion and respect for human dignity.* The Woodstock group proposed that a new social covenant should affirm that patient care is the primary goal and responsibility of the system. It is unethical for the health care provider to exploit the vulnerability of the patient in order to enhance the organization's or a professional's income or profits.

- *Commitment to professional competence.* Health care professionals, including physicians, executives, and trustees, have an ethical responsibility to continue their education and enhance their competence in a given field.

- *Commitment to a spirit of service.* Health care professionals have a responsibility to the community they serve as well as to individual patients. One important way in which this spirit is demonstrated is by providing uncompensated or undercompensated care to the poor and needy.

- *Honesty.* Health care professionals have an ethical obligation to maintain accurate and truthful medical records, including information provided to third-party payers. Patients and families should receive honest information about their clinical condition as well as the costs of care.

- *Confidentiality.* Information about the patient should be shared only with express permission of the patient or legal guardian, except as required by law.

- *Good stewardship and careful administration.* Health care professionals have an ethical obligation to use common resources wisely, thinking carefully about the relative costs and benefits of treatments.[3]

After agreeing on the core principles, the Woodstock participants identified the five most common and broadly defined types of ethical dilemmas faced by professionals in the business aspects of health care:

1. When resources are inadequate to meet needs;
2. When providers own or profit from patient utilization of specific services;
3. When rules or regulations conflict with professional judgement;
4. When truthfulness may be in conflict with patient confidentiality; and
5. When patients' own behavior contributes significantly to their problems.

They then applied the core principles in an attempt to provide guidance on how they should be addressed ethically. Although unanimity was not obtained as to the best approach in every instance, the group was able to generally reach consensus in most areas. Finally, the Woodstock seminar participants developed "checkpoint" questions that individual professionals can use in responding to the most frequent ethical dilemmas they face in the business of health care. An example of several such "checkpoints" for ethical decision making is included in Table 3-1, page 71.[3]

Table 3-1
Checkpoints for Ethical Behavior

When the needs of my patients or community exceed my capacity to provide uncompensated or undercompensated care:

- Have I made an effort to solicit resources from others in my community to support additional uncompensated care?

- Have I advised my patients about my limits and helped to direct them to other sources?

- Have I set priorities among the patients who come to me in ways that are consistent with my mission statement and based on medical need and potential benefit, without regard to such factors as race, gender, lifestyle, economic status, or age, except where such factors are medically relevant?

Whenever the rules and regulations of third-party payers conflict with my professional judgment:

- Have I provided the third-party payers with appropriate and relevant information about my patient's presenting conditions, actual services I have performed for my patient, my recommended treatment path, and the patient's progress?

- Have I made a good faith effort to understand the spirit and purpose of the rules or regulations, so that I can seek a compromise that responds to my patient's needs?

- Have I informed the patient about the conflict, and about the various treatment options available, and invited the patient to participate in a resolution?

In the course of ordinary record keeping and billing:

- Am I careful to record fully all relevant medical information in my patients' medical records?

- In billing third-party payers, am I scrupulously honest about reporting services I actually perform?

When patients' behavior contributes significantly to their problems:

- Do my personal views on my patients' behavior lead me to withhold care from them that is medically required or to deny them attention or respect?

- Am I treating patients with respect while counseling them on the destructive nature of their behaviors and helping them find ways to change those behaviors?

Whenever I am troubled by the decisions or actions I am taking:

- If, after careful reflection, I am uncertain about whether a certain action is ethical, have I consulted with a respected colleague or other appropriate professional?

- If I am repeatedly troubled by a specific regulation, procedural requirement, expectation, or practice that colleagues seem to have accepted as appropriate, have I sought ways to challenge that practice, to substitute a more ethically acceptable procedure or practice, or at least to bring the issue up for debate and discussion?

Source: Woodstock Theological Center: *Ethical Considerations in the Business Aspects of Health Care.* Washington, DC: Georgetown University Press, 1995. Used with permission.

Organization Ethics in Professional Codes and Joint Commission Standards

The Joint Commission's preamble statement on patient rights and the American Hospital Association's (AHA's) "Statement on a Patient Bill of Rights" in the 1970s were among the first documents that delineated a health care organization's ethical responsibility to its patients. Throughout the 1980s and continuing in the 1990s, many health care organizations have developed mission, vision, and values statements as well as codes of professional ethics or conduct to set forth the guiding ethical principles and values of the organization.[4]

In its 1992 Management Advisory entitled "Ethical Conduct for Health Care Institutions," the AHA affirmed the unique ethical responsibilities of health care organizations:

> Health care institutions, by virtue of their roles as health care providers, employers, and community health resources, have special responsibilities for ethical conduct and ethical practices that go beyond meeting minimum legal and regulatory standards. Their broad range of patient care, education, public health, social service, and business functions is essential to the health and well-being of their communities. These roles and functions demand that health care organizations conduct themselves in an ethical manner that emphasizes a basic community service orientation and justifies the public trust. The health care institution's mission and values should be embodied in all its programs, services, and activities.[5]

Professional societies and associations, including the American Medical Association, American Nurses Association, National Hospice Organization, and American Psychiatric Association, as well as many others, have also published codes of ethics governing professional behavior of their members which address some components of organization ethical behavior. The Code of Ethics of the American College of Healthcare Executives, for example, addresses the executive's responsibilities to the profession of health care management, to patients, to the organization, and to the employees. The code also addresses real or potential conflicts of interest, and states

> The executive shall:
>
> ■ Conduct all personal and professional relationships in such a way that all those affected are assured that management decisions are made in the best interests of the organization and the individuals served by it;
>
> ■ Disclose to the appropriate authority any direct or indirect financial or personal interests that pose potential or actual conflicts of interest;
>
> ■ Accept no gifts or benefits offered with the express or implied expectation of influencing a management decision; and
>
> ■ Inform the appropriate authority and other involved parties of potential or actual conflicts of interest related to appointments or elections to boards or committees inside the health care executive's organization.[6]

What areas should the scope of organization ethics encompass and through what mechanisms? The Rights and Ethics function in each Joint Commission accreditation manual requires that the health care organization develop and implement a framework, code, or practices that support an ethical environment for the patients as well as for the community served. Areas that an organization will want to consider in meeting these standards include developing manager and staff conflict-of-interest policies, organization mission and value statements, and policies addressing how integrity in clinical decision making will be maintained despite financial incentives to the organization or individual practitioners. The standards and intents provide guidance regarding the major areas that should be addressed in any organization ethics code or framework.

Strategies for Addressing Organization Ethics

If we think of ethics as What is the right thing to do? or What is the good? we clearly see that ethical decision-making confronts the health care manager or practitioner on a regular basis in everyday practice. An ethical organization is proactive in its approach to integrating values and principles into the daily operations of the organization. In addition to formal ethics mechanisms such as committees or consultants, the ethical life of a health care organization is lived in a diverse set of structures and processes, including mission and values statements, administrative policies and procedures, financial processes, marketing materials and advertisements, human resource practices, and daily leadership activities. Conflicts and dilemmas of a crisis nature, often of the sort faced in clinical ethics case consultation, can be minimized through policies and structures that are founded on deeply held organization values such as integrity, trust, stewardship, and honesty. Table 3-2 (page 74) provides examples of the scope of policies, activities or processes that a health care organization may wish to address as components of a multifaceted framework of organization ethical behavior.

Developing and Implementing an Ethical Infrastructure

How should a health care organization approach the development of an ethics framework that supports moral leadership and practice within the organization? Because each health care organization is unique in its scope of service, history, sponsorship, and relationship to the community, it would be difficult to suggest a single formula that would fit every possible situation or type of organization. However, even given the range and diversity of health care organizations, David Renz and William Eddy of the University of Missouri-Kansas City Bloch School of Business and Public Administration propose a basic ethics infrastructure for health care organizations that summarizes innovative approaches used by corporations such as Unisys, US West, and 3M. The basic ethical infrastructure

- has an organizational systems orientation and a linked set of structures and processes;
- focuses on the entire range of ethical issues and decisions, including individual, professional, and institutional issues;
- is responsive to the ethical standards of all stakeholders to the institution, including the community and its diverse constituencies;
- has taken a long-term perspective; and
- involves all levels of the organization, including board members, health care professionals, patients and families, executives, and representatives of the broader community.[7]

Table 3-2

Sample Components of an Organization Ethics Framework

- Organization mission, vision, philosophy and values statements
- Publication or distribution of ethics standards and mission and values statements to the community
- Mechanisms for receiving and using public feedback about the ethical performance of the organization
- Use of community members on governing bodies and advisory committees with explicit mandate to monitor the ethics of the organization
- Conflict-of-interest policies for the governing body, senior managers, and staff
- Corporate compliance plan for fraud and abuse prevention and monitoring
- Financial management, reimbursement, and billing policies and practices
- Human resource management policies for staff selection, promotion, confidentiality of employee information such as salary and health status, transfer, disciplinary action, harassment, benefits, and termination
- Policies rewarding exemplary ethical behavior in the organization, as well as handling violations discreetly and respectfully
- Policies addressing the ethical use of financial incentives for managers, physicians, and staff while ensuring integrity in clinical decision making
- Accurate marketing representation of the organization's scope of services, hours of service, fees, admission criteria, and relationships with other organizations
- Discharge planning practices, especially if the patient is referred to another service of the organization
- Referral relationships with other organizations or practitioners
- Relationships with vendors
- Policies governing admissions and the transfer of patients to other organizations
- Policies on acceptance of gifts or cash
- Information management policies which protect patient confidentiality
- Codes of conduct addressing personal and professional boundaries between patients and staff
- Policies on solicitation of donations from patients, families, vendors, and the community
- Administrative policies and organization practices which ensure compliance with applicable law and regulation
- Strategic planning initiatives that consider community needs and just resource allocation
- Grievance mechanisms
- Institutional Review Board (IRB) policies and procedures
- Partnership and joint venture agreements
- Marketing and advertising plans
- Policies governing the relationship of the organization to affiliated organizations, including educational institutions

On the basis of successful change processes in other businesses, Renz and Eddy suggest four practical strategies for implementing this infrastructure or framework:

1. Conduct a formal process to clarify and articulate the organization's values and link them to the mission and vision;

2. Facilitate communication and learning about ethics and ethical issues, including values clarification and reflection on their link to practice;

3. Create structures that support and encourage a culture of ethical integrity; and

4. Create processes to monitor and offer feedback on ethical performance.[7]

Using this model, a health care organization might begin the process of designing a framework for organization ethics by developing and communicating statements of organization mission and values with the input of leaders, staff, physicians, patients, and the community served.

Developing and Implementing an Organization Mission and Values Statement

Documents such as mission and values statements, developed through organizationwide discourse and revised periodically, can often stimulate organizations to base their actions on these carefully depicted relationships, values, and traditions.[4] Larger health care organizations sometimes find that forming a multidisciplinary committee or task force, comprising several governing body members, senior managers, clinicians, and administrative and support staff, is an effective way of drafting a mission and values statement that represents a cross-organization perspective. In smaller organizations, leaders might seek staff input in drafting an organization values statement through such techniques as brainstorming and multivoting. Such processes can serve to organize informal practices and assumptions into an effective organization statement that provides guidance in both business and clinical decision making. Many organizations include their mission, vision, and values statements in organization literature such as patient brochures, annual reports, new employee orientation programs, and employee handbooks.

Many religious or faith-based health care organizations express their long-standing traditions of compassion, commitment to the poor, and stewardship in their mission, values, or philosophy statements. Figure 3-1 (page 76) includes an example of such a philosophy statement from Provena Mercy Center in Aurora, Illinois. Another example document in Figure 3-2 (page 77) presents an integrated mission, vision, and values statement from Rainbow Hospice, Inc, a community-based hospice organization located in Park Ridge, Illinois.

Facilitating Learning About Ethics and Values Clarification

Once the mission, vision, and values statements have been developed and distributed to patients, employees, physicians, and the community, the health care organization faces a great challenge in clarifying their intent and linking these statements to daily practice. It is often helpful for the organization to provide practical and understandable examples of how the values are expressed in the actions of leaders and staff toward patients and toward each other. For example, a health care organization that espouses fairness as one of its values might present an

Figure 3-1	Statement of Philosophy
	Provena Mercy Center

Believing in the value and call of this ministry, we at Mercy Center for Health Care Services strive to

- serve persons of all religious beliefs, mindful of the healing gospel of Jesus Christ;
- provide a high quality environment where patients and their families will find that all hastens good health care;
- work together as health care providers;
- foster communication, education, empowerment, and excellence;
- attend to each person's diverse and changing physical, emotional, social, and spiritual needs;
- value each patient's right to make responsible decisions about treatment alternatives;
- exercise prudent stewardship of human and financial resources;
- collaborate with local constituencies that support the patient's ongoing healing processes; and
- advocate for social justice.

This organization statement of philosophy expresses the religious values at the core of their ministry.

Source: Provena Mercy Center, Aurora, Illinois. Used with permission.

example of how the organization's "fairness in billing" statement incorporates this value in the organization's financial practices. An employee grievance policy in which staff members of the organization are given the opportunity to appeal what they perceive to be an unfair performance appraisal is another such example of how the value of fairness can be implemented in human resource management. Leaders and staff should be oriented to the policies and practices that support the established ethical framework, and this education should be updated at periodic intervals when changes occur.

Creating Structures to Encourage an Ethical Culture

Building on the foundation of the organization's mission and values statements, some health care organizations have further expressed their commitment to fostering an ethical culture by developing structures such as conflict-of-interest policies, ethical standards, and codes of professional conduct. These documents are often useful in giving explicit guidance to staff and leaders on ways to incorporate ethical decision making in maintaining appropriate practitioner-and staff-patient relationships as well as in daily business activities such as contracting or purchasing supplies and equipment from vendors. When properly implemented, they can provide important and useful structures by which ethical values such as honesty or stewardship are woven into the organization's culture and daily operations.

Figure 3-2	**Mission, Vision, and Values Statement**
	Rainbow Hospice

Our Mission: Rainbow Hospice enables people to live with dignity and hope while coping with loss and the end of life.

Our Vision: Our vision is to be Chicagoland's foremost provider of palliative care, to be a vital resource for education and to enrich the lives of those we serve.

Our Values:

- *Excellence:* To continually challenge ourselves to do better.

- *Honor and Respect:* To honor the dignity and worth of each individual and to respect the breadth of cultures, values, and traditions.

- *Compassion:* To be present for others without judgment offering hope, comfort, and support.

- *Commitment:* To work together as we actualize our mission and to be ethical in all that we do.

This integrated mission, vision, and values statement represents the ethical principles of this hospice organization.

Source: Rainbow Hospice, Inc, Park Ridge, Illinois. Used with permission.

Advocate Health Care, a large health system based in the greater Chicago metropolitan area, expanded upon its five core values—equality, compassion, excellence, partnership, and stewardship—in an organization ethics statement that publicly expresses how the values will guide the organization's behavior in the activities of patient care, billing, marketing, and external relations. The statement was prepared by a cross-organization task force comprised of staff directly working in the activities highlighted above. The Advocate Health Care Ethics Statement is included as Figure 3-3 (pages 78 and 79). Another example of a code of ethics, one developed by community-based Hospice of Boulder County, includes the organization's core values and provides specific examples of how they are implemented in practice (see Figure 3-4, pages 80 through 82).

Leader and Staff Conflicts of Interest

In the past, an organization policy addressing the disclosure and avoidance of a potential or actual "conflict of interest" was applied almost exclusively to governing bodies and senior managers, yet this concept applies to all staff and practitioners within the health care organization. Management conflicts of interest often relate primarily to financial interests or management decisions in contracting, whereas staff conflicts of interest may be a result of competing or dual interests or commitments to the organization, the patients or families served, their own financial self-interest, and other organizations and the community.

In long term care, home care, and hospice organizations, the risks for potential conflicts of interest for staff are often the result of close or long-standing relationships that are formed, as between the residents and the aide staff of a nursing home. In home care and hospice organizations, this risk is heightened

Figure 3-3	Ethics Statement
	Advocate Health Care

Preamble

Advocate Health Care's five values—equality, compassion, excellence, partnership and stewardship—are an expression of organizational as well as personal beliefs and convictions. In this Statement we publicly profess how our values will guide our organization's behavior in four areas of organizational activity—patient care, billing, marketing, and external relations. (Future versions may address additional areas of organizational behavior.) This Statement will assist us in weighing our values and choosing among alternative courses of action in decision and policy making. As a living expression of Advocate's values, the Statement is a work in progress. The Advocate community is asked to study and examine the Statement and to participate in the process of continuing review and revision.

Ethics in Patient Care

*Guided by our value of **compassion***

■ We will care for patients throughout the continuum of care on the basis of medical judgment and with due consideration for their personal preferences.

*Guided by our value of **stewardship***

■ We will care for patients throughout the continuum of care in the context of our commitment to responsibly manage available resources.

*Guided by our value of **equality***

■ We will formulate timely and appropriate patient care plans in conjunction with the patient, the family and/or significant others, and members of the health care team.

*Guided by our value of **partnership***

■ We will provide to our associates and other care givers appropriate information—including the patient's follow-up treatment plan, explanation of medication and medical equipment, and advance directives—as patients are transferred within the continuum of care

Ethics in Billing

*Guided by our value of **excellence***

■ We will issue accurate, understandable, and timely bills to patients and payers and charge only for services rendered.

■ We will interact with our customers through associates who are well informed about the billing process and responsive to inquiries and requests for assistance in this process.

Ethics in Marketing

*Guided by our value of **excellence***

■ We will protect the confidentiality of our customers and associates who participate in research or other information-gathering forums.

*Guided by our value of **partnership***

■ We will exercise responsibility in communications with external and internal audiences and avoid misleading or exaggerated statements.

(continued)

Figure 3-3	Ethics Statement
(continued)	Advocate Health Care

*Guided by our value of **equality***

■ We will create communications that are responsive and sensitive to our diverse audiences and seek the opinions of our customers and associates in developing our communications.

Ethics in External Relations

*Guided by our value of **partnership***

■ We will select partners who promote values and business practices consistent with ours.

■ We will promote partnerships with community-based organizations in an effort to benefit our local communities.

*Guided by our value of **equality***

■ We will conduct our relations with partners in a way that promotes diversity and avoids discrimination and unfair treatment.

*Guided by our value of **excellence***

■ We will strive to contain costs while continuously improving the quality of our services.

■ We will expect all our associates to avoid foreseeable conflicts of interest in external relationships and we will work collaboratively with them to remove actual or potential conflicts of interest.

*Guided by our value of **stewardship***

■ We will manage the resources entrusted to us and our partners in a responsible, accountable, and environmentally sound manner.

Approved by the Advocate Health Care Board of Directors on September 20, 1995.

This detailed ethics statement of Advocate Health Care provides specific examples of how the organization's core values are implemented in practice in four areas of activity—patient care, billing, marketing, and external relations.

Source: Advocate Health Care, Oak Brook, Illinois. Used with permission.

because the staff are interacting with patients and families outside the structure of an institution in the patient's place of residence. Elderly patients with few family supports may view the home care or hospice staff and volunteers as "surrogate" family members, and may begin to relate to the staff accordingly by giving them gifts, requesting their assistance in financial decision making, calling on them for inappropriate services, and sharing intimate information about their lives which is unrelated to their health care. In behavioral health organizations, staff conflicts of interests are sometimes related to the development of inappropriate personal relationships with patients or clients receiving care, a serious therapeutic as well as ethical concern.

Sometimes the issue may appear so insignificant or harmless to staff that they fail to recognize the inherent conflict of interest within it. One example might be a

Figure 3-4 | **Code of Ethics**
Hospice of Boulder County

Introduction

The vision of Hospice of Boulder County is to serve all persons living with terminal illness, their families, their caregivers, and those affected by death and dying in the community; to support patient comfort, dignity and choices; to be a leading resource in clinical, ethical, and spiritual issues of dying and grief; and to create partnerships with other providers in response to the changing health care environment.

In order to ethically, effectively, and sensitively meet the needs of each other and of those whom we serve, we have developed this Code of Ethics. We, the staff and volunteers of Hospice of Boulder County, hold these core values to be integral to our mission and our aim will be:

Core Values

Respect

Clients and their support people

- To honor choices that are made regarding care and treatment
- To be sensitive to variations in cultural, spiritual, religious, ethnic, or lifestyle values
- To maintain absolute confidentiality, except as dictated by the need to communicate within the team and with respect for imminent danger to self or others

Within Hospice of Boulder County

- To be sensitive to variations in cultural, spiritual, religious, ethnic or lifestyle values
- To respect the right of staff to refuse an assignment that challenges their personal or moral values
- To maintain confidentiality as it relates to performance issues, pay, and personal issues
- To respect the skills and limitations of each employee and to empower them to succeed

Within the community

- To maintain confidentiality as it relates to issues within HBC
- To uphold the reputation of other community agencies and care providers, but would address ethical and sub-standard care issues
- To maintain confidentiality of businesses and agencies with whom we work

Integrity and Honesty

Clients and their support people

- To fully disclose information related to treatment options or care choices
- To accurately represent the services offered by hospice
- To refrain from inappropriate or intimate relationships with those we serve
- To avoid the acceptance of gifts

Within Hospice of Boulder County

- To create an environment in which staff and administration can have open and honest communication

(continued)

Figure 3-4	Code of Ethics
(continued)	**Hospice of Boulder County**

- To provide an honest appraisal of job performance and suggestions and guidelines for improvement
- To have honest exchanges between peers with regard to work related issues
- To ensure that staff are qualified and competent to perform assigned functions

Within the community

- To create honest working relationships with other agencies, facilities, care providers, vendors, and payers
- To exercise honesty in marketing and fund development activities
- To make and obtain referrals that are in the best interest of those we serve

Caring

Clients and their support people

- To identify and endeavor to meet the needs of family members and significant others as well as those of the patient
- To affirm and support caregivers in their efforts

Within Hospice of Boulder County

- To recognize and endeavor to meet the support needs of co-workers
- To recognize and celebrate accomplishments

Within the community

- To engage in educational and public awareness offerings that promote the appropriate use of hospice and grief support services
- To create programs that meet the needs of those in the schools, churches and workplaces
- To provide individual and group counseling

Fair and Equitable Allocation of Resources

Patients and their support people

- To respect the admission criteria of payer sources in order to respect their resources
- To not make decisions related to admission or treatment of patients based on financial reasons alone
- To provide care based on patient and family need
- To provide services regardless of the ability to pay
- To consider the survival of the agency in making decisions

Within Hospice of Boulder County

- To provide a competitive compensation and benefit package
- To be fair in scheduling and allocation of the work load
- To provide an adequate physical work space
- To offer assistance and encouragement for on-going education and personal growth

(continued)

Figure 3-4	Code of Ethics
(continued)	Hospice of Boulder County

Within the community

■ To be honest in the solicitation of financial support from the community, businesses and foundations

■ To utilize funds according to the wishes of the donors and in accordance with local, state and federal regulations

■ To provide counseling, education and support to the community regardless of remuneration

■ To expand services to meet the needs of unique populations or the under-served

Approved by the Ethics Committee of Hospice of Boulder County, 1996

A hospice developed this code of ethics to meet the needs of the organization and of those they serve. The code is built on the core values of respect, integrity and honesty, caring, and fair and equitable allocation of resources.

Source: Hospice of Boulder County, Longmont, Colorado. Used with permission.

home care nurse who identifies that a wheelchair-bound patient needs a ramp built to the front door in order to safely leave the home. The nurse then suggests to the patient that the nurse's relative, a carpenter, could construct the ramp for what the nurse represents as a "reasonable" fee. The nurse may perceive this "referral" as only being helpful to a patient with limited resources and a fixed income; however, another perspective might interpret the action as the nurse using her knowledge of the patient's situation and vulnerability to benefit a relative's business as a carpenter. The patient, not wanting to appear ungrateful to the nurse for her interest and recommendation, may feel pressured to hire the nurse's relative for fear of retribution or interruption in the nurse's services. This scenario reflects a potential conflict of interest between the nurse's professional role and relationship to the patient and the nurse's familial relationship to the carpenter whom she is recommending.

In its code of ethics, the American College of Healthcare Executives defines a conflict of interest as existing whenever a health care executive either acts to benefit himself or herself directly or indirectly (for example, through a friend or relative) by using authority or inside information, or when the individual uses authority or information to make a decision that intentionally affects the organization adversely.[6] Table 3-3 on page 83 provides examples of the common types of conflicts of interest faced by governing body members and senior managers. A health care organization may want to address these in its written policies and procedures, administrative processes, and codes of ethical conduct. As described earlier, physicians, clinicians, and other staff of the organization might also be faced with situations that present a conflict of interest between their primary responsibility to the well-being and best interest of the patient and some other value or interest. Table 3-4 on page 84 provides examples of the kinds of real or potential conflicts of interest that a health care organization may want to consider when drafting policies and procedures for clinical staff, including physicians.

Table 3-3

Examples of Potential Conflicts of Interest for Health Care Managers

- Entering into business relationships that are likely to conflict with the organization's mission and values statements related to patient or resident care

- Conducting organization business with a firm that employs or is controlled by a relative or close associate

- Using information gained from serving on the board of a community agency to develop a competing service

- Owning a business (for example, an organization cleaning service) that does business with the health care organization where the manager is employed

- Using organization resources (for example, supplies, clerical support, equipment, patient lists) for one's own personal gain, such as for starting a new business or serving on a professional board

- Sharing or selling "trade secrets" or proprietary information from the organization with a competitor or outside entity

- Accepting gifts, gratuities, or discounts from vendors that might influence management decisions (for example, entertainment, cash, material personal gifts, loans)

- Disclosing confidential information (for example, sensitive financial information, legal actions, computer access codes, strategic planning documents) about the organization to outside parties

In its Management Advisory titled "Resolution of Conflicts of Interest," the AHA recommends that health care organizations develop a written policy on conflicts of interest with two primary objectives in mind:

- to assure the good faith and integrity of its officers, governing body members, administrative staff, including physicians in that role, and employees; and

- to provide a systematic and ongoing method of assisting individuals in disclosing and resolving conflicts of interest.

The advisory includes specific examples of disclosure and resolution statements, as well as a questionnaire for leaders and employees to disclose any potential conflict of interest.[8]

Creating Processes to Monitor and Provide Feedback on Ethical Performance

The final strategy for building an ethical infrastructure suggested by Renz and Eddy is the creation of processes to monitor and offer feedback on the organization's ethical performance. Provena Home Health Care, based in Frankfort, Illinois, approached this strategy through a planned process that included a staff-needs assessment, education on the organization's business ethics standards, and follow-up monitoring. The organization gathered information on the staff's views of the ethical climate of the organization approximately two weeks before its first ethics and values training, (see Figure 3-5, page 85) and then repeated the same survey several months after the training sessions for a comparison. In the first survey, many staff responded that "ethics" did not apply to them or that they were by

Table 3-4

Examples of Potential Conflicts of Interest for Practitioners and Staff

- Making clinical or therapeutic decisions about patient care based on the potential profit, incentives, or financial benefit to the individual or organization

- Self-referring by a practitioner to another organization or service in which the practitioner holds a financial interest

- Soliciting of private business from patients and families (for example, a home health aide seeking private employment with the patient for off-hours work)

- Accepting of significant gifts or cash from patients and families

- Violating professional boundaries with patients and families (for example, health care professional serving as durable power of attorney for patient, managing a patient's or client's financial affairs, dating a patient or client or his/her family member)

- Sharing confidential information about the organization with outside parties

- Making referrals (for example, a discharge planning referral) based on inducements from an outside organization (for example, a home care organization) or an individual financial interest in the outside entity

- Making contractual arrangements with vendors or suppliers (for example, an enterostomal therapist who is on retainer from a product manufacturer to encourage patients to use the supplier's products without informing patients of other available and competing products)

- Fee-splitting for referrals to another practitioner or organization

- Accepting of loans from patients, families, or vendors

nature ethical people and therefore did not need this training; however, subsequent surveys revealed a much greater discernment of the nuances of ethics that arise in everyday life within the organization. As a component of the training, a corporate *Standards of Business Conduct* booklet, in which the Provena Health's core values and business practices are highlighted, was shared with staff. The booklet's statement of purpose is included as Figure 3-6 (page 86). Some of the standards of conduct covered in this guide include the following:

- Service and customer satisfaction, such as relationships with vendors and conflicts of interest;

- Awareness and respect for others, including confidentiality of information, patient autonomy, and staff rights;

- Open communication and managerial relationships; and

- Simplicity and management by fact, such as accurate reporting of data and use of resources.[9]

Corporate compliance plans frequently delineate mechanisms by which the organization will monitor itself against predetermined indicators of ethical business practices, codes of conduct, and law and regulation. In September 1994, Price Waterhouse conducted a comprehensive survey of approximately 60 Fortune 250 companies in an effort to learn more about those strategies that are successful in implementing corporate compliance plans. The survey identified

Figure 3-5	Values Survey
	Provena Home Care

Instructions

This survey is designed to assess your Home Health department's ethical standards. Please respond to the questions honestly and candidly. Your responses will be kept confidential.

1. Do you understand the organization's values and ethical expectations?

❏ Yes ❏ No ❏ Somewhat

2. Do you feel that your organization "practices what they preach?"

❏ Yes ❏ No ❏ Somewhat

3. Do your organization's rules for doing business stay the same in good times and when things are not going well?

❏ Yes ❏ No ❏ Somewhat

4. Is the organization's ethical code of conduct as important as financial goals?

❏ Yes ❏ No ❏ Somewhat

5. Are your organization's ethics considered in day-to-day decision making?

❏ Yes ❏ No ❏ Somewhat

6. Do you understand the consequences for violations when you make ethical decisions?

❏ Yes ❏ No ❏ Somewhat

7. Do you receive positive feedback from management when you make ethical decisions?

❏ Yes ❏ No ❏ Somewhat

8. Do you receive positive feedback from coworkers when you make ethical decisions?

❏ Yes ❏ No ❏ Somewhat

9. Are you expected to apply ethical guidelines to every aspect of your job?

❏ Yes ❏ No ❏ Somewhat

10. Do you feel you can approach anyone in management and raise an ethics question?

❏ Yes ❏ No ❏ Somewhat

11. Is there training available to help new employees understand the ethics and standards of the organization?

❏ Yes ❏ No ❏ Somewhat

This survey is designed to assess staff's views of the ethical climate of the organization. It was conducted approximately two weeks before the first ethics and values training and then repeated several months after the training sessions for a comparison.

Source: Provena Home Care, Frankfort, Illinois. Used with permission.

Figure 3-6	Standards of Business Conduct
	Provena Health

Purpose

To Reflect Our Mission: This booklet was designed to help us make good business decisions because our mission is reflected in all we say and do. These standards apply to:

- all employees
- anyone who acts on our behalf in any way

You Are Responsible: You are responsible for the results of the decisions you make. When questions arise, it is your job to ask for help. Talk to your supervisor and utilize the Standards of Business Conduct, many of which are described within this booklet.

You may face situations in which you must make difficult decisions. Your actions should be guided by these standards, as well as your own personal standards. Before you make a decision, you should ask yourself the following questions:

- Is this decision legal?
- Does it comply with our policies?
- Is it consistent with our Mission and Values?
- If my decision were made public, how would I feel?
- Would I advise family or friends to make this decision?

IF YOU DON'T KNOW...ASK!

The Guidelines: Our Values provide the guidelines that help us live our Mission. Our Standards of Business Conduct are based on these Values. They help to define what is allowed, and what is not allowed in our daily business activities. These Values are reflected in a passage from the Old Testament book of Micah. In Chapter 6, verse 8(b) reads,

And what does the Lord require of you?
To act justly and to love tenderly
and to walk humbly with your God.

The statement of purpose from a booklet outlining one corporation's standards of business conduct is shown here. As a component of ethics training, the entire booklet was shared with staff to highlight the core values and business practices of the organization.

Source: Provena Health, *Standards of Business Conduct.* Used with permission.

certain companies whose proactive and innovative approaches exceeded the minimum requirements necessary for meeting law and regulations. Price Waterhouse determined these programs to be "leading edge." One of the key characteristics in the leading-edge companies was the strong leadership commitment to setting an organization tone that discourages employee wrongdoing and detects improper conduct. These programs were also based in a commitment to ethical values and exemplary conduct (integrity based) rather than a list of dos and don'ts (rule based) which often fails to address root causes of misconduct. Leading-edge programs codified their compliance policies in an easy-to-understand document that addresses all areas of compliance, including conflicts of interest and ethical business practices.[10]

The Visiting Nurse Association and Hospice of Northern California, a large home health and hospice organization based in Emeryville, California, developed a comprehensive compliance program addressing administrative, financial, and clinical components of the organization. Key indicators in these areas are monitored through the corporate compliance plan under the direction of the board of trustees (see Figure 3-7, pages 88 and 89). Many of these indicators encompass compliance with operational protocols that are designed to prevent fraud and abuse in billing and referrals practices, including physician referrals, payment for physician oversight of the patient's plan of care, verification of all visits submitted for reimbursement, and other business practices. Employees are encouraged to identify and report questionable business practices without fear of reprisal, and follow-up investigations are documented, analyzed, and used to formulate changes in operational policies and practices (see Figure 3-8, page 90).

Nurturing an ethical climate in any health care organization is a challenging task. Leadership commitment and role modeling are essential to raising the awareness of organization ethics issues as well as the strategies and processes to address them. The next chapter will address assessment approaches as well as example educational plans and resources that help to further manager and staff awareness and knowledge of both clinical and organization ethics and decision-making approaches.

References

1. Lyman RL: From clinical ethics to organizational ethics: The second stage of the evolution of bioethics. *Bioethics Forum* 12(2):3–12, 1996.

2. Schyve PM: Patient rights and organization ethics: The Joint Commission perspective. *Bioethics Forum* 12(2):13–20, 1996.

3. Woodstock Theological Center: *Ethical Considerations in the Business Aspects of Health Care.* Washington, DC: Georgetown University Press, 1995.

4. Reiser SJ: The ethical life of health care organizations. *Hastings Cent Rep* 24(6):28–35, 1994.

5. American Hospital Association: Ethical conduct for health care institutions. *AHA Management Advisory* pp 1–3, 1992.

6. American College of Healthcare Executives: *Code of Ethics.* Chicago: American College of Healthcare Executives, 1995.

7. Renz DO, Eddy WB: Organizations, ethics, and health care: Building an ethics infrastructure for a new era. *Bioethics Forum* 12(2):29–39, 1996.

8. American Hospital Association: Resolution of conflicts of interest. *AHA Management Advisory* pp 1–5, 1990.

9. Provena Health. Standards of business conduct. Apr 1997.

10. Pell G: Corporate compliance programs: Leading edge practices. *Corporate Conduct Quarterly* 5, 1997.

Figure 3-7	Corporate Compliance Plan Monitors

Visiting Nurse Association and Hospice of Northern California

Standard of Conduct	Specific Monitor	Rationale	Methodology
Education of appropriate staff on laws and regulations governing job duties	Staff are oriented to the laws and regulations governing their job duties; and then routinely trained on any changes or additions to those regulations	**High Risk:** Fraud/Abuse COP/Title XXII	Review of orientation materials per job class and education log, department inservice and/or information distribution
Patient rights and responsibilities	Patients informed of their rights and responsibilities *prior* to initiation of care (100% of admissions)	**High Risk:** COP/Title XXII	Chart review and supervisory visits
Patient participation in plan of care	Documented patient/family participation in POC	**High Risk:** COP/Title XXII	Random chart review and supervisory visit
Patient safety	Safety assessments completed on all patients	**High Risk:** COP/Title XXII	Random chart review
Patient grievance and/or complaints	Patient/family complaints will be handled per HHA protocol and aggregated for possible trends	**High Risk:** COP/Title XXII	Staff and managers education and review of complaint file and/or log
Staff competency	All staff will have credentials and references verified at time of hire: Licenses and certifications must be current and a copy verified and on file; home health aide competencies will be verified at time of hire	**High Risk:** COP/Title XXII	Review of clinician employee file and independent contractor/ registry files
One level of care	All patients are provided services according to acceptable standards of care and physician orders	**High Risk:** COP/Title XXII	Random review of charts
Supervision of home health aides	All patients with home health aide services are supervised, per policy, every two weeks (under skilled service POC)	**High Risk:** COP/Title XXII	Random review of charts
Acceptable practice standards	All clinical staff adhere to professional practice standards (e.g., all home health aides follow care plans as assigned by RN or therapist)	**High Risk:** COP/Title XXII	Random review of charts
Payment for referrals	No payment will be made by HHA for patient referrals	**High Risk:** Fraud/Abuse	100% review of all contracts by legal staff
Personal referrals for patient services	All employees shall refrain from recommending or placing business with companies in which they have a personal interest and/or other benefit	**High Risk:** Fraud/Abuse	Staff education and adherence to HR policies
Employees should not recommend hiring of close family members	Employees should not be working in close proximity with family members, especially in a managerial/subordinate position	**High Risk:** Fraud/Abuse	Staff education and adherence to agency hiring policies
Acceptance of gifts (if gift implies an obligation on part of recipient)	No employee shall accept gifts from any organization that currently conducts business with, or wishes to conduct business with the HHA. No gifts will be accepted from anyone, if it is implied that there is a reciprocal obligation	**High Risk:** Fraud/Abuse	Staff education and adherence to HR policies and standards of conduct

(continued)

Figure 3-7	Corporate Compliance Plan Monitors
(continued)	VNA and Hospice of Northern California

Standard of Conduct	Specific Monitor	Rationale	Methodology
Loyalty and appearance of conflict of interest	All employees shall review their conduct to make sure they are supportive of the HHA and no appearance of conflict of interest exists	**High Risk:** Fraud/Abuse	HR policies and staff education
Employee employment that conflicts or interferes with the mission of the HHA	No employee may be employed by another HHA (if that HHA interferes with, or competes with own HHA) without permission of management	**High Risk:** Fraud/Abuse	HR hiring policies and staff education
Personal use of HHA property	No property will be used for personal purposes without the express permission of the HHA manager and/or administrator. All employees shall treat HHA property with respect and protect it from deterioration.	**High Risk:** Fraud/Abuse	Staff education and HR policies
Employee use of HHA assets	No employee may utilize HHA time, assets, facilities, materials, influence for charitable activities without express written permission of senior management and copy shall be retained in employee file.	**High Risk:** Fraud/Abuse	Staff education and HR policies
Employee ownership conflict of interest	No employee shall own or have direct interest in a competing agency with HHA	**High Risk:** Fraud/Abuse	HR policies and staff education
Contract(s) legality	All contracts conform with appropriate federal state, and/or local laws	**High Risk:** Fraud/Abuse	100% review of all contracts by legal
Plan of care	Physician orders (POCs) generated within agency timeframes, signed by physician and dated and filed in record within 20 business days	**High Risk:** COP/Title XXII	Review of POC list and random audit of clinical records
Patient bills and record accuracy	Accurate and timely invoices (visits/supplies) verified against patient clinical record notes and physician orders. No bills submitted (Medicare) before signed order back in chart	**High Risk:** Fraud/Abuse	Random review of invoices of patient records
Records and logs maintenance	All patient records and/or other records that are covered by applicable state, federal, and/or agency policy are maintained per such policy	**High Risk:** COP/Title XXII	Random review of filing status
Confidentiality of patient records	All records pertaining to individual patients should be treated as confidential by all staff, even following discharge from the HHA	**High Risk:** COP/Title XXII	Staff education during orientation and at periodic intervals
Organizational performance improvement plan	IOP is effective in documenting HHA performance improvement	**High Risk:** COP/Title XXII	Review of plan, processes and current programs to quantify outcomes
Periodic review of HHA administrative and clinical policies and procedures	Annual review of policies and procedures	**High Risk:** COP/Title XXII	PAC minutes of review and recommendation process

One large home health and hospice organization monitors key indicators addressing administrative, financial, and clinical components of the organization. This form tracks the standard of conduct, specific monitor, rationale (including risk and Medicare Conditions of Participation), and method of monitoring established by the board of trustees. COP, Medicare Condition of Participation; HHA, home health agency; HR, human resources; IOP, improving organization performance; POC, plan of care.

Source: Visiting Nurses Association and Hospice of Northern California, Emeryville, California. Used with permission.

Figure 3-8	Corporate Compliance Report Form

Visiting Nurse Association and Hospice of Northern California

Reporting Individual:	Date of Report:
Office/Department Where Incident Occurred:	Date of Reported Incident:

Description of Incident Reported:

_____
_____
_____

Standard of Conduct:

❏ Patient Care and Comfort   ❏ Law and Regulations

❏ Business Conduct and Practices   ❏ Conflicts of Interest   Specific Area: _____

Investigation Warranted:

❏ Yes   ❏ No   If No, Rationale for Decision: _____

_____

_____

Investigation Report:

_____

_____

_____

_____

_____

Date Reported to COC *(within 72 hours of investigation)*: _____

Recommendations Accepted by COC: ❏ Yes   ❏ No

Follow-up Actions Suggested:

_____

_____

_____

_____

_____

_____

Policy/Protocol Change _____   Institute as Monitoring Indicator: ❏ Yes   ❏ No

Investigation and/or report to Board of Trustees: ❏ Yes ❏ No   Date: _____

Signature of person completing this report: _____
_____

This compliance report form allows employees to identify and report questionable business practices and documents the investigation and follow-up actions.

Source: Visiting Nurses Association and Hospice of Northern California, Emeryville, California. Used with permission.

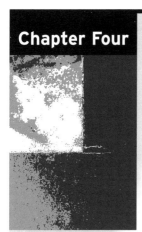

Chapter Four

Designing and Implementing a Framework for Clinical and Organization Ethics

A framework or mechanism for addressing patient rights and clinical and organization ethics should be multidimensional and based on the size, scope, resources, and needs of the health care organization and the patients or residents it serves. As with the design or redesign of any process or function, it is often useful to begin with a baseline assessment of the organization, so that structures and education can be developed in accordance with the organization's objectives and goals. For example, a large, university-affiliated medical center will have very different needs from those of a student health clinic or a long term care facility. A large organization may find a formal ethics committee structure as well as a consultation service necessary to address the myriad of ethical concerns that arise both in patient care and in organization operations. On the other hand, a small community-based home health agency may not identify the need for a committee per se, but rather may design an ethics framework consisting of staff training, policies and procedures, and discussion of ethical concerns at staff meetings and patient case conferences. Similarly, a behavioral health organization providing residential treatment services to an adolescent patient population may incorporate its ethics mechanism into existing processes such as multidisciplinary team treatment planning and administrative and clinical protocols or policies and procedures. However, regardless of the size and scope of the organization, it is essential that the organization incorporate ethics awareness and knowledge into the existing clinical and organization processes.

Any health care organization, regardless of size, scope, or available resources, may find the following questions or issues a useful starting point in designing and implementing its ethics framework or mechanism:

- What is the level of knowledge of leaders and staff about patient or resident rights and ethics in general? Are staff able to differentiate an ethical concern or conflict from a patient or resident complaint, compliance with law and regulation, or a public relations issue?

- What training is provided to leaders and staff about patient or resident rights and ethics?

- What processes are currently in place to address patient or resident rights and ethics, including patient or resident rights documents, a mission and values statement, policies and procedures, codes of professional conduct, an ethics committee, ethics consultation, and staff training?

- What processes are in place to address staff rights and values, such as requests to be relieved from certain patient care responsibilities because of an ethical, philosophical, cultural, or religious conflict?

- Do leaders and staff know how to access the existing mechanisms? How often are they used and for what purposes?

- Do patients, residents, families, and the community have access to the existing ethics mechanisms, when appropriate?

- Is there a model used for ethical decision making that incorporates ethical theory, principles, or values rather than merely basing decisions on personal opinion or emotion?

■ What resources are available for initial and ongoing training and reference, such as published codes of ethics, books, journals, access to ethics centers or consulting ethicists, "grand rounds" discussions on ethics topics, or training videotapes?

■ Is there alignment between the published organization policy and what happens in actual practice? If not, where are there discrepancies, and why?

■ Is there a mechanism by which leaders and staff can sort out their own values and determine how these are influencing their judgments?

Conducting a Baseline Assessment

By starting with a baseline assessment of the effectiveness of any existing structures as well as leader and staff understanding about ethical principles and values, the organization can better determine its training needs as well as design structures to integrate ethics and values into daily practice. Unless training is provided, many staff may fail to recognize ethical values, principles, and conflicts as they occur, and thus their ability to discern an appropriate course of action may be impaired. An awareness of ethics and values needs to be a vital part of the daily business of the organization, not something prepared for external reviewers or simply to meet the "letter of the law." For example, organizations that provide written information at admission about the patient's right to formulate an advance directive should also ensure that the appropriate staff understand its intent so that patient and family questions can be completely and accurately answered. Knowledge of applicable law and regulations, such as the Patient Self-Determination Act, cannot be confined to the ethics committee or the risk-management department of the organization—all staff should have knowledge appropriate to their position and job responsibilities within the organization, especially if they are dealing directly with patients or residents.

Some health care organizations have found that a formal assessment process such as the one available through the Educational Development Corporation (EDC), "Decisions Near the End of Life," is useful for both starting and enhancing an ethical framework within the organization. This educational program, developed by EDC in conjunction with The Hastings Center, consists of two parts: an assessment phase followed by a multilevel educational process. In the assessment phase, organization staff complete a comprehensive questionnaire that examines beliefs and attitudes about life-sustaining treatments, determines knowledge about medical ethics (including guidelines and legal standards), identifies organization impediments to good decision making in the use of life-sustaining treatments, and assesses patient and family satisfaction regarding their involvement in such decisions. Questionnaire results are summarized by the EDC and the organization receives a profile of their knowledge base, which can then be used to plan staff training. The second phase of the program includes additional training in which the results of the profile are discussed and selected ethical issues are explored in more detail.[1]

At Iowa Lutheran Hospital (Des Moines), a baseline assessment conducted in 1994 using the EDC process served as the foundation for a long-term educational plan generated by the organization's ethics committee. The last question asked on their 70-question survey, which was completed by approximately 300 staff (including physicians), was "How knowledgeable do you consider yourself to be about basic principles and issues in medical ethics?" This question received a mean response of only 2.65 on a scale of 1 to 5, with 1 representing "Not knowledgeable", 3 representing "Somewhat knowledgeable," and 5 representing "Very knowledgeable." The results of the assessment, or institutional profile, helped the leadership team design a series of small group educational modules to educate the staff on issues that represented the strongest learning needs. Iowa Lutheran intends to conduct a second survey of its staff in 1998 to assess the outcome of its educational initiatives.[2]

Other organizations have used less formal processes for determining baseline needs. One approach might include the distribution of a confidential survey to all staff and volunteers, asking for input on the design and role of an ethics committee as well as suggestions for educational topics ranging from advance directives to patient confidentiality to professional codes of conduct. When this has been done, some organizations also elicit staff feedback regarding the kinds of ethical concerns that they face in daily practice. One home care organization that used a confidential survey as a baseline assessment experienced a very high response rate and identified numerous ethical challenges that had never before risen to the surface for discussion and policy development. Examples of the kinds of issues raised by staff included the extent of their professional responsibility to patients and families who live in unsafe environments, working with patients who are non-compliant with their established plan of treatment, responding to terminally ill patients who indicate an intent to hasten their deaths through medication overdose, and dealing with conflicts between the patient, physician, and the organization. This type of information is extremely valuable in setting the course of the organization's ethical journey, especially with respect to staff knowledge and educational needs.

Designing and Implementing an Ethics Education Plan

For knowledge about ethical values and decision making to become fully integrated throughout the organization rather than remain strictly the purview of an ethics committee, the organization must equip its leaders and staff, including physicians, with educational resources based on their assessed learning needs. Education must also consider the beliefs and values that these individuals bring as part of their own life experience and personal philosophy. It is important to distinguish among the educational needs of various constituencies: the needs of a newly formed ethics committee or consultation team will be somewhat different in scope and depth than those of an "ethics awareness" training for all staff. For example, members of an ethics committee that will determine policy for the organization, as well as offer recommendations on difficult clinical cases, may require more in-depth study on ethical theory, decision-making models, legal standards and precedents, and the organization's existing policies and procedures. Committee members often receive this type of training through attending intensive ethics courses or seminars or through training provided by a consulting ethicist. On the other hand, certified nursing assistants in a long term care facility may have educational needs focused more on topics such as respect for resident autonomy within a community setting, resident confidentiality, end-of-life decision making, and the organization's policy on the safe use of chemical or physical restraints. Providing or arranging for this kind of education based on assessed needs is often a key role that ethics committees serve.

As the discipline of bioethics has evolved over the past 30 years, its study has moved out of universities and into health care organizations, professional societies, national and international conferences, and bioethics centers. In the early 1990s, The Hastings Center embarked on a consensus project to determine what should comprise the basic curriculum for any serious student of bioethics. Project participants, representing universities and ethics centers from around the country, identified these six key areas for education:

1. The history of medical ethics and bioethics;

2. Theoretical foundations and methods of analysis, including religious traditions, philosophical theories, and the nuances of moral argument;

3. Comparative analyses and scope of the issues encompassed by the term bioethics, including areas such as end-of-life decision making, the Human Genome Project, and international health issues;

4. Moral issues of professionalism, including the patient-professional relationship;

5. Cultural contexts of bioethics; and

6. Resources in the field, including leading books and journals.

The Hastings Center concluded that the goal of bioethics education should be for students to acquire the ability to apply the knowledge in making "real life" as well as theoretical decisions.[3] A health care organization might want to focus on only selected areas from this or other suggested topic lists, based on what are the most important issues for its community or scope of service.

Health care organizations vary greatly in their approaches to bioethics education, from extensive training for ethics consultants and committee members to case discussions in staff meetings. The University of Chicago Hospitals has designed a comprehensive and multifaceted educational plan called Integrated Ethics that bridges the efforts of the University of Chicago's MacLean Center for Clinical Medical Ethics, The University of Chicago Hospitals, and the University of Chicago Pritzker School of Medicine. The goal of the Integrated Ethics program is to coordinate outreach in clinical medical ethics to medical students and medical residents as well as a multidisciplinary mix of physicians, nurses, social workers, chaplains, and therapists, as well as others involved in direct patient care. Rooted in a belief that adult learners learn in different ways and through different educational approaches based on their individual needs and interests, the range of educational offerings provided includes free-form discussion and support groups, topic-based discussions, videos, and articles. Among the many topics that have been addressed are communication and listening skills, professional boundaries, medicine in literature, ethnic and cultural differences, delivery of difficult news,

Table 4-1

Integrated Ethics Program: University of Chicago Hospitals

- *Ethics consultations*, both formal and informal, which serve as a teaching tool in daily practice

- *Multidisciplinary ethics team*, which includes staff who serve as resources in identifying the need for staff education and in raising staff awareness regarding the need for an ethics consultation

- *Unit-specific ethics focus groups*, which raise issues and often lead to policy development or revision and provide an opportunity to practice effective communication strategies

- *Multidisciplinary Ethics Teaching Case Conferences (METCC)*, the most popular form of ethics education, which provide an opportunity to discuss difficult cases and ethical dilemmas in a non-threatening and multidisciplinary environment

- *Project "Ponder This…"*, which encourages respondents to ponder situations and two or three process-oriented ethical questions distributed by e-mail

- *Brown bag* lunches and discussion on medical ethics in the media for multidisciplinary staff and medical students

- *Discussions on issues surrounding death and dying* for staff and medical students

- *New staff hospital orientation*, which includes an introduction to clinical medical ethics and patient rights

- *Overview of clinical medical ethics* and orientation on how and when to call an ethics consultation

- *Orientation on advance directives* for new social workers

- *Orientation to ethical issues related to the care of hospice patients*, which is required for general medicine multidisciplinary staff and those caring for hospice patients

- *Orientation to ethical decision making in the neonatal intensive care unit*, as well as annual updates

- *Orientation to ethical issues surrounding domestic violence* for multidisciplinary staff and medical students

- *Participation of medical ethicist* in weekly or biweekly unit-based patient care conferences

Source: Camille Renella, RN, Clinical Medical Ethicist, The University of Chicago Hospitals. Used with permission.

personal values clarification, the meaning of suffering, the meaning of life and death, religious or faith differences, staff or physician error or fallibility, and organization ethics. Integrated Ethics is intended to offer a broad range of opportunities to foster ethical reflection and participate in focused discussions on a wide variety of ethical issues as they impact on patient-centered care; educational approaches include the use of vignettes, role-play, inservices, and the development of patient/family teaching tools, among others.[4] Table 4-1 (above) represents a listing of the various approaches and topics included in the Integrated Ethics framework.

The Ethics Outreach Services of the Loyola University of Chicago's Center for Ethics has designed an 18-session course by which the Center's consultants pre-pare ethics committees of health care organizations for independent functioning at the completion of the program. The first 12 sessions include a lecture followed by a directed discussion working out the ethical issues of a case on the basis of the concepts developed in the lecture. The aim of these sessions is for ethics com-mittee members to develop a common base of understanding that the group can use in their eventual deliberations. In the second series of six educational sessions, the consultant leads the committee in discussing actual or hypothetical cases, for the purpose of the committee's ongoing education and opportunity to apply new learning. The consultant also assists the organization in developing structures and processes for referral of cases to the committee. Table 4-2 (page 99) includes a summary of the curriculum design for the first 12 educational sessions.[5] The table represents a training course for a home health/hospice organization, but can be adapted for any health care organization's ethics committee training.

Another university-based clinical ethics program, the University of New Mexico Health Sciences Center Ethics Program, has developed a listing of seven core com-petencies in clinical ethics, as well as specific examples of evidence. The seven competencies and behaviors highlighted in Table 4-3 (page 100) represent exam-ples of core competencies in clinical ethics which may be helpful in designing an educational plan and defined competencies in an acute care setting. Many organi-zations find that the most effective training in ethics awareness for staff is that which is grounded in day-to-day realities within the organization, whether those issues concern patient care dilemmas or organization policies and codes of con-duct. Many ethics centers, consultants, reference services, and educational resources are available throughout the country. Many of those that have been use-ful in designing relevant and organization-specific training programs, both for staff and ethics committees, are included in the Resources on page 129. Organizations are encouraged to explore various alternatives for ethics training, including resources and case study examples now available on the Internet from a number of bioethics centers.

Provena Home Care (Frankfort, Ill) has developed a basic four-hour ethics awareness training program for all clinical and support staff which uses case dis-cussion, videotaped exercises in ethical decision making, and examination of simple, practical ethical questions that are commonly experienced by staff in prac-tice. The goal of the training is to provide a basic conceptual framework and a common language for discussion of ethical issues, particularly those dealing with organization ethics or staff conduct, and to promote a workplace of integrity. Staff are encouraged to raise ethical concerns in an open and nonthreatening environment. Figure 4-1 (page 101) provides an example of a simple clinical scenario which staff are asked to analyze in the context of organization ethics.

Ethics education for the long term care staff at Lifelink, (Bensenville, Ill) a health and human service organization, includes many of the practical and every-day types of ethical concerns that staff face when caring for a geriatric resident

Table 4-2

Ethics Committee Training Program: Loyola University of Chicago Center for Ethics

- *Ethics Committees:* The typical functions and charge of this committee, experience to date of ethics committees in health care organization settings, the health care ethics community and its literature and organizations, and a primer on how to discuss ethics cases and sample cases for discussion.

- *Process of Ethical Decision Making:* Basic concepts of ethics and ethical decision making, role-based obligations and the ethical commitments deriving from the organization's mission, addressing conflicts between alternate bases of obligation, and sample cases for discussion.

- *Alternative Approaches to Ethical Decision Making—Part 1:* Values-maximizing and rule- based moral thinking, as well as sample cases discussed from each of these points of view.

- *Alternative Approaches to Ethical Decision Making—Part 2:* Rights-based and virtues-based moral thinking, the role of story/narrative/context in ethical decision making, and sample cases discussed from each of these points of view.

- *Ethical Concepts and Decision Making by Competent Patients:* Informed consent and other models of caregiver-patient relationship and sample cases to discuss.

- *Ethical Concepts and Decision Making for Patients with Diminished or No Capacity to Participate:* The role of other decision makers in such decisions, widely accepted principles to guide these situations and difficulties in applying them, and sample cases to discuss.

- *Central Values of Home Health and Hospice:* Issues of clarity, ambiguity, and conflict, admission criteria, patients and families who do not fully comply, and sample cases to discuss.

- *Home Health and Hospice Values as These Interact with Other Values Systems in Health Care:* The role of values and the mission of the specific organization, dealing with conflicts between different sets of values, and sample cases to discuss.

- *Ethical Distribution of Health Care Resources:* Approaches to questions about justice and rights regarding access to health care resources, concepts and issues in macrorationing (designing a just system of health care), and sample cases to discuss.

- *Ethical Concepts and Issues about Microrationing:* Rationing of specific health care resources for fixed populations who need them and sample cases to discuss.

- *Ethical Concepts and Issues in Relation to Managed Care:* The current system of distribution and the ethical concerns and conflicts that it raises and sample cases to discuss.

- *The Role and Obligations of the Case Consultant and the Case-Consulting Committee:* Aims and appropriate outcomes for effective case consultation and sample cases to discuss.

Source: David Ozar, PhD, Director, Loyola University of Chicago Center for Ethics. Used with permission.

Table 4-3

Clinical Ethics Competencies: University of New Mexico Health Sciences Center

■ *Professional Responsibility:* Assume responsibility for the profession as a whole, understand emergency treatment duties, do not harm, do not abandon patients, understand one's own biases, provide for continuity of care, keep abreast of important research and changing practice standards, understand rights and duties of both patients and professionals, and understand one's own limitations.

■ *Patient Rights:* Understand autonomy and informed consent, obtain valid consent or refusal of treatment, understand medical and legal dimensions of decisional capacity, know how to proceed if treatment is refused, and understand appropriate use of ethics committees and consultants.

■ *Privacy and Confidentiality:* Understand how to protect patient privacy as well as duty to inform, inform patients on limits of confidentiality, and understand legal requirements of reporting.

■ *Truth-Telling:* Tell the truth, and understand those specific circumstances when it might be morally justified to withhold or delay information.

■ *Reproductive Ethics:* Understand ethical and legal issues of reproductive decision making, including abortion, birth control, sterilization, sexually transmitted diseases, reproductive research, genetic screening and counseling, treatment decisions for seriously ill neonates.

■ *Distributive Justice:* Understand issues of access and barriers to health care, alternative models of equitable delivery, individual rights and the public good, impact of technology, and managed care.

■ *Research Ethics:* Understand ethics and the law of research on humans as well as animals, informed consent, patient care or comfort versus research imperatives, access to new therapeutic research treatments, use of placebos, conflicts of interest, and duty to share research results.

Source: University of New Mexico Health Sciences Center Ethics Program. Used with permission.

population, including dealing with the hostile resident, sexuality in nursing homes, nursing ethics, and end-of-life decision making.[6] Other long term care facilities find that gearing the ethics education to the common scenarios that confront residents and staff is a useful educational design. For example, a long term care facility might have little need to focus on organ procurement policies, whereas education on how to determine appropriate limitations on resident autonomy within a community setting (for example, how to set meal, bath, and sleep times) might be essential.

Designing and Implementing Mechanisms for Addressing Rights and Ethics

The Joint Commission's Rights and Ethics standards require that the health care organization establish a defined process or mechanism for addressing both clinical and organization or business ethics. Although ethics committees or consultation teams per se are not required by the Joint Commission's accreditation

Figure 4-1	Clinical Scenario Worksheet

Provena Home Care

Mary, in her work as a CNA, has become "friends" with Mrs. Jones. During her visits, Mary begins to share more information about herself and her difficulties with her boyfriend. Mrs. Jones offers to "help."

1. What type of standard or ethical dilemma would this be?_____
_____

2. Utilizing the quick test, what is the impact on the organization and individuals involved?_____
_____

3. What should the CNA do in this situation? _____
_____

4. What is our organization's philosophy pertaining to this type of situation? _____
_____

5. How frequently does this happen?

Never	Rarely	Often	Common Practice
1	**2**	**3**	**4**

_____

This sample clinical scenario is used in a home health ethics awareness training. CNA, certified nurse assistant.

Source: Provena Home Care, Frankfort, Illinois. Used with permission.

standards, many health care organizations find these structures extremely useful in reviewing and resolving specific clinical cases representing difficult ethical challenges as well as in developing or reviewing organization policies in both clinical and organization ethics. Some larger health care organizations and health networks or systems have developed a role of "ethics officer" or function of "mission integration" as other mechanisms to address organization ethics. Smaller organizations with a more circumscribed scope of services, such as a behavioral health residential center, an ambulatory clinic, or a home medical equipment supplier, may not identify a need for a separate ethics committee, and may instead choose to integrate the concepts of ethical decision making into existing organization structures such as staff meetings, management retreats, multidisciplinary team planning meetings, and case conferences.

When forming or revitalizing an organization ethics committee, it is helpful to begin with analyzing the data gathered during the baseline assessment phase of formation, and as described earlier, to follow this with programs to meet the assessed educational needs of the committee members. The organization will also want to consider the membership, roles and responsibilities, scope of inquiry, and access to the committee in this development phase. Table 4-4 (page 102) includes a listing of questions to consider before establishing the committee. Many of the same questions should be asked if and when an ethics consultation service is formed that is separate from that of the committee role. In larger health care organizations where there may be multiple avenues of ethical discussion and case

Table 4-4
Questions to Consider When Forming an Ethics Committee

- How will committee members be selected? What types of experts are needed (for example, physicians, attorneys, nurses, therapists, ethicists, chaplains, social workers, dietitians, pharmacists, paraprofessional staff, managers, and community members)?

- How often will the committee meet?

- Who should have access to the committee and through what avenues? How will this access be communicated throughout the organization? Who determines which issues or cases the committee reviews?

- What are the initial and ongoing educational needs of the committee?

- How will the roles and responsibilities as well as the scope of the committee functions be defined in written policy?

- What will be the role of the committee in developing, reviewing, and approving policies and procedures for the organizations (for example, do-not-resuscitate policy, withdrawal of life-sustaining treatment)?

- What role will the committee have in providing education to other staff in the organization?

- What will be the role of the committee in case consultation? How will the committee prepare for a case consultation?

- What model or methodology will the committee use in providing case consultation?

- What relationship will the committee have to other ethics mechanisms in the organization, such as a consulting ethicist or ethics consultation team?

- How will the committee communicate its recommendations?

- How will the committee's work be documented? Should case consultation be documented in the patient or resident record?

- How should the confidentiality of the committee's activities be addressed?

- Will the committee consider both clinical as well as organization ethical concerns?

- How will the committee assess its effectiveness?

consultation, it is beneficial to define the goals and objectives, scope, and skills required by the individuals involved in each structure or process.

Rush-Presbyterian-St Luke's Medical Center in Chicago has a multidimensional ethics framework, including an Ethics Consultation Service. At its affiliated home care organization, Rush Home Care Network, the Ethics Education and Consultation Consortium serves as the organization's mechanism for considering ethical issues that arise in patient care and provides education and consultation to staff. The consortium consists of the medical center's consulting ethicist as well as multidisciplinary staff representatives who are interested in and educated on ethical decision making. The consortium meets bimonthly to consider specific cases and offer educational sessions to staff. In addition, the consortium provides "stat" or priority consultation for cases of immediate concern. Figure 4-2 (page 103) describes a referral flow for the stat consultation process. The consortium

Figure 4-2 Stat Ethics Consultation Flowchart
Rush Home Care Network

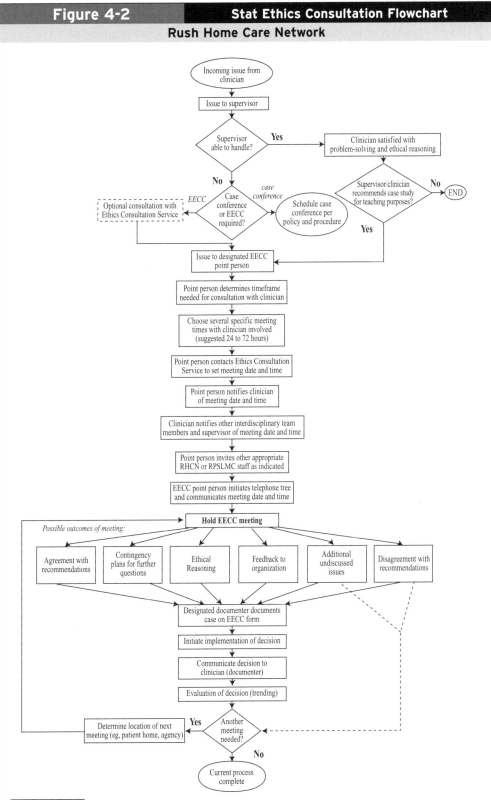

This flow diagram outlines the process for a staff member requesting an urgent consultation for an identified ethical concern. EECC, Ethics Education and Consultation Consortium.

Source: Rush Home Care Network, Chicago, Illinois. Used with permission.

documents its discussion and recommendations on a discussion summary form, included as Figure 4-3 (page 105).

Mayo Medical Center in Rochester, Minnesota, has both an ethics committee and a 40-member ethics consultation team, whose multidisciplinary members undergo an extensive training program in order to equip them with the consultation skills necessary to respond to requests for complex case consultations. When an ethics case consultation is requested, several members of the team respond to provide more than one point of view. One of the keys to the success of this mechanism has been the active involvement and support of a number of physicians representing various specialties who serve as consultation team members. The Mayo Medical Center's ethics consultation service is highlighted in Figure 4-4 (pages 106 through 108).

An important function for the ethics committee or consultation service includes providing education to staff and others on their role and the process for accessing their services. Methodist Hospital (St Louis Park, Minn) distributes a brochure to staff and patients advising them of the services of the Biomedical Ethics Committee (see Figure 4-5, page 109). Similarly, The University of Chicago Hospitals distributes an educational brochure to its staff (see Figure 4-6, pages 110 and 111) outlining common concepts in ethical reflection, such as advance directives and informed consent, as well as the process for accessing a formal or informal ethics consultation.

Evaluating the Effectiveness of Ethics Mechanisms

With the rapid development of ethics committees and consultation services in many health care organizations in recent years, ethicists have identified a need for closer scrutiny and self-evaluation of the effectiveness of these mechanisms. An ad hoc committee of the Kansas City Regional Ethics Committee Consortium, in conjunction with the Midwest Bioethics Center, developed a self-assessment tool for ethics committees. The tool is intended to generate questions and discussion among the committee members that will be useful in directing future activities of the group, especially in the areas of committee operations, educational responsibilities, case review, and policy development. This self-assessment tool is included as Figure 4-7 (pages 112 through 115).

Other organizations have found it useful to periodically survey staff and leaders of the organization to elicit their feedback about the effectiveness of existing ethics mechanisms as well as to determine their ongoing educational needs, values, and attitudes. Whatever the blend of evaluation techniques used by the organization, it is essential that the established structures and processes serve a useful purpose in enhancing the organization's ethical awareness and level of reflection.

Going Through a Joint Commission Survey

During an actual accreditation survey, the surveyors use a variety of evaluation approaches to determine whether the organization has effectively met the requirements of standards in the Rights and Ethics chapter as well as other applicable chapters.

Figure 4-3	Ethics Discussion Summary Form

Rush Home Care Network

Date of Request:	Consult Date:	Case #

Initiator of Request: _____
❏ staff   ❏ patient   ❏ family   ❏ physician   ❏ supervisor   ❏ other

Receiver of Request: _____
❏ on-call   ❏ peer   ❏ supervisor

Issue: _____

Principals
❏ Staff_____ ;   _____
❏ Patient/family _____ ;   _____
❏ Other_____

Nature of Concern: _____

EECC Recommendations for Plan of Action: _____

Ethical Issues: _____

Referrals Made To: _____

Outcomes (What effect did recommended actions have? Situation improved? etc):_____

Evaluation of Outcomes: _____

Date Reviewed by EECC:_____

Additional Evaluation/Comments: _____

Statistical Data
Response Time from Request to Initial Response: _____ hours
On-call Peer Member Needed Assistance from:
❏ ethicist   ❏ social worker   ❏ external community resource
❏ no one   ❏ clinical nurse specialist or supervisor   ❏ other_____
❏ psychiatric nurse
Case Conference Called: ❏ Yes   ❏ No   Date/Time: _____
In attendance:

_____   _____
_____   _____
_____   _____

Documenter/Recorder: _____
_____

This form provides a simple summary of an ethics consultation and discussion.

Source: Rush Home Care Network, Chicago, Illinois. Used with permission.

Figure 4-4	Hospital Ethics Consultation Service
	Mayo Medical Center

Philosophy Statement

The primary responsibility for medical care and resolution of ethical problems in patient management lies with the physician, the health care team, the patient, and the patient's family. The physician/patient relationship should be protected from outside intervention to the fullest extent possible. The purpose of the Mayo Medical Center Hospital Ethics Consultation Service is not to interfere with that relationship, but to facilitate it to the greatest extent possible. Our goal is to review difficult situations and the options available to the health care providers and the patients or their surrogates. It is the expressed intent of the Hospital Ethics Consultation Service that the consultations be entirely advisory and in no way legislative or binding.

Service Composition

The Hospital Ethics Consultation Service consists of individuals representing the disciplines of medicine/surgery, nursing, Social Services, Chaplaincy, Administration, and legal affairs (ex-officio). One member of the Consultation Service will be on call at a given time with the on-call tour of duty being one week. That individual will provide the initial response to a request for consultation, and then convene from the core group a working subcommittee to help address each consultation request. At least one physician and one nurse, and one representative from Administration, Social Services, and/or Chaplaincy should be present for the discussion of the discussion of the case. It is desirable to have legal counsel present for the discussion, but if this is not possible then the case should at least be discussed on the telephone with one of our members from the Legal Department. It is the goal of the Service to provide a multidisciplinary review of each situation, bringing to bear multiple points of view and expertise in resolving the ethical dilemma. This multidisciplinary approach will also provide a framework of checks and balances, ensuring that no one point of view is imposed upon the situation.

Consultation Procedures

Initiation

Requester referred to Hospital Ethics Consultation Service (HECS) via operators

Triage

- Is the issue an ethical dilemma? What is the question?
- If a complaint, refer to patient representative or administration.
- If a legal question only, refer to legal.
- If requester is not staff physician, has the requester discussed the concern with staff? If not, why not? In general we should encourage individuals to try to solve the problem themselves. Only after such an effort has taken place will we get involved.
- If the issue is an emergency and can't wait for a full consultation, talk the individual through the problem. If you have questions, call or refer the requester to the appropriate staff.
- If consultation declined or if contact was only a question, dictate a brief memo describing the contact and forward to Administration.

(continued)

Figure 4-4	**Hospital Ethics Consultation Service**
(continued)	**Mayo Medical Clinic**

Preliminaries

If someone other than the primary physician (or his surrogate) requests the consultation, page the consultant to let him/her know of the request. Get his/her perspective and understanding. Set up a time to meet if interested.

Notify the head nurse of the patient's unit of the request. Similarly, obtain perspective(s) and set up a time to meet and interview the patient's primary nurse(s).

Data Collection

Review and abstract the medical record. Use the Consultation Worksheet (additional copies can be obtained through Administration).

Interview all pertinent individuals, always include staff, nursing, the patient and/or his/her surrogate. Give family members an opportunity to speak with you, the consultation team. *Always see the patient.*

Data Collected:

- *Medical Indications:* The medical facts—the diagnoses and treatments employed. What are the goals of treatment(s)?

- *Patient Preferences:* Does the patient have decision-making capacity? If not, who is the surrogate? What does the patient/surrogate want? What are her/his goals? Does s/he understand what is happening or recommended? Is there an advance directive? Is the surrogate operating under substituted judgment or the best interest standard?

- *Quality of Life:* What are the potential outcomes of the interventions(s) or lack of intervention? In what shape will the patient arrive. Are the outcomes consistent with the goals and values of the patient?

- *Contextual Features:* Are there other issues that are important to the case: legal concerns, ethical principles, social context, religious beliefs, emotional and financial considerations, family and other relationships, etc.

Scheduling

Establish a location for the consultation meeting. Usually this is a conference room closest to the patient's room. Reserve room use.

Contact other service members and arrange for a meeting of a working quorum (usually to convene between 4:00 and 5:30 pm).

Quorum: Physician - 1, Nurse - 1, Legal - 1 (if a member from legal cannot attend, at least call one of the members to discuss the case), Administration, Social Services or Chaplaincy - 1.

Inform all interested and necessary individuals of time and location of meeting.

Meeting

The medical record must be present at the meeting.

The on-call individual will present the case to the team and assembled guests.

All individuals who wish to speak to the group may do so. After all interviews are complete all but the consultation service members will be excused to allow free and open discussion.

(continued)

Figure 4-4	Hospital Ethics Consultation Service
(continued)	Mayo Medical Center

The goal is to provide review of a given question or provide ethically appropriate options.

All recommendations are advisory.

Conclusion

Call and notify the requester and any and all appropriate individuals of the conclusion(s).

Write a consultation note in the medical record, briefly listing the question(s), the conclusions and those facts and reasoning that underlie the conclusions.

Complete the consultation worksheet. The worksheet and/or a dictated summary should be submitted to Administration.

If possible, obtain feedback from the requester or other individuals about how the case was handled, suggestions for improvement, etc.

Follow-up

As much as possible, follow the case to see ultimately what happens—implementation of recommendations, disposition of patient, etc.

When the report is received in Administration an evaluation form will be sent to the requester and others involved for feedback.

If there are ever any questions call appropriate staff.

This procedure is used by an ethics consultation service to facilitate the resolution of ethical problems encountered in medical care.

Source: Mayo Medical Center, Rochester, Minnesota. Used with permission.

Document Review

One component of the survey is the review of policies and procedures as well as other documents related to this function. Depending on the type of organization and its scope of services, this document review might include

- patient or resident rights and responsibilities documents;

- policies and procedures regarding advance directives, withholding resuscitation, withdrawing or foregoing life-sustaining care or treatment, and end-of-life care (including pain and symptom management);

- written policies and procedures for conducting research or investigational studies, organ donation and procurement, patient or resident confidentiality, and the organization's complaint investigation mechanism;

- written policies and procedures for patient or resident informed consent, decision-making capacity, advocacy, guardianship, or protective services;

- organization policies and procedures related to appropriate admission, billing, transfer, discharge, and marketing practices;

- written descriptions of the organization's relationship to other health care providers, educational institutions, and payers;

Figure 4-5	Biomedical Ethics Committee Brochure

Methodist Hospital

What is the Biomedical Ethics Committee?

Patients come to Methodist Hospital with a range of concerns. In most situations, decisions about what treatments are best are relatively clear, but in some cases questions may arise. When questions arise, the Biomedical Ethics Committee at Methodist Hospital is available to assist patients, family and the health-care team in understanding the ethical issues which may be of concern.

The Biomedical Ethics Committee is comprised of a multidisciplinary team including physicians, nurses, chaplains, social workers, hospital staff and community members. Family, patients, staff or anyone with an ethical concern can seek assistance either from individual committee members or from the entire committee.

What is an ethical concern?

The way in which we, as individuals, see ourselves is determined by our beliefs and principles. These principles guide our choices about how we relate to each other individually, as a community, and spiritually. Sometimes, these principles conflict with medical decision-making.

Ethical concerns in medical care arise from differing goals, beliefs and perspectives.

What are some of the ethical concerns in health care?

- How should machines and therapies be used in the treatment of patients, even when the patient's condition cannot be reversed?
- When there is disagreement among family members or within the health-care team about the appropriate course of treatment.
- The health-care team and family are fairly certain of a decision, but still feel uncomfortable and would like to explore it further.
- A recommendation for treatment conflicts with a patient's or family's religious beliefs.
- A treatment may save the patient's life, but the patient will continue to have severe problems or disabilities.
- The patient is suffering: What else can be done? What else should be done?
- Patient and family disagree with the health-care team about the appropriate course of treatment.

How do I make a request for an ethics consultation?

Family, physicians and other health care professionals may request an ethics consultation through the patient's physician, the nursing staff or by phone:

- During regular working hours the request can be made through the Medical Staff Office at **555-5135.**
- During off-hours and on weekends, the request may be made by contacting the Nursing Supervisor at **555-5000.**

The Biomedical Ethics Consultation Service is offered at no charge.

This information is provided to patients and families to educate them about the biomedical ethics resources available to them.

Source: Methodist Hospital, St Louis Park, Minnesota. Used with permission.

Figure 4-6	**Clinical Medical Ethics Brochure**
	University of Chicago

Clinical Medical Ethics: It's more than just a DNR status!

1. Who should consider having an **advance directive?**

2. If a patient refuses a physician's order for a treatment **who decides?**

3. What four questions could you ask a patient to help determine his/her **decision making capacity** (DMC)?

4. What constitutes **informed consent?**

5. What is your obligation when patient report is being conducted in the middle of the hall?

6. What is the difference between a **formal** and **informal** Ethics Consultation?

7. What is the procedure for calling an ethics consultation?
   Who initiates it?
   When should a consult be called?
   Where do you find the protocol for calling if?

Answers

1. *Every* patient should consider having an **advance directive.** The patient and physician should have ongoing discussions about the patient's wishes before there is a crisis in care and these discussions should be documented as they occur.

2. Before this question can be answered, several preliminary questions must be considered, including: Does the patient have Decision Making Capacity? Has a surrogate decision maker been appointed by the patient? Does the patient have an Advance Directive? What are the benefits vs. burdens of care to the patient? In any case, the patient has the right of Self Determination which includes Health Care Decision Making. See Administrative and Nursing Policies and Procedures for additional information.

3. **Decision making capacity** criteria:
   a. What is your main medical problem right now?
   b. What treatment was recommended for **this** problem?
   c. If you receive or do not receive **this** treatment what will happen?
   d. Why have you decided to receive (or not) receive this treatment?
      (Assess if consistent with patient's own values.)

4. **Informed consent** means that the patient has been given sufficient information so that he/she understands the nature of the treatment, the risks, consequences and probability of success of the proposed procedure, the alternatives, and prognosis if the procedure is not performed or any treatment given. It is the responsibility of the physician to ensure that informed consent is appropriately documented and a progress note describing all informational exchange between the physician and patient should be written in the patient's medical record.

5. In order to protect **patient confidentiality,** it is your **obligation** to move the discussion/report to a secluded area, away from patients, families, and other hospital personnel.

6. **Formal ethics consultation:**
   a. requires the knowledge and approval of the patient's attending physician,

(continued)

Figure 4-6	Clinical Medical Ethics Brochure
(continued)	University of Chicago

b. a note of consultation including recommendations **will be** entered into the patient's chart,

c. the case **will be** presented at the Ethics Case Conference at the Center for Clinical Medical Ethics (CCME).

Informal ethics consultation:

a. the attending **may** or **may not** be involved in the discussions,

b. unless a patient or family called the consult, the Consultant **will not** talk with the patient or family, and they need not
be made aware that a consult was called,

c. a consult note **will not** be written in the patient's chart,

d. the case **will not** be presented at Case Conference at the CCME (unless especially selected for teaching purposes).

7. According to the **protocol** located in all the policy and procedure manuals, Ethics Consultations are conducted to address patient care situations that present complex medical, ethical and/or legal issues which warrant further discussion and/or clarification. This service is available 24 hours per day, 7 days per week.

All attending physicians, house staff, patients and families can call a **formal** or **informal ethics consultation.** To do so, just:

a. page the Clinical Medical Ethics Fellow on call, page #0522, **or**

b. contact the Clinical Medical Ethicist in Patient Services at 0-3813 or pager #0571, **or**

c. call the University of Chicago Center for Clinical Medical Ethics, 0-1453.

All other staff can call a **formal** or **informal** consult by contacting the Clinical Medical Ethicist in Patient Services at 0-3813 or pager #0571.

This information is made available to staff to provide additional guidance during both formal and informal ethics consultations.

Source: The University of Chicago Hospitals, Chicago, Illinois. Used with permission.

- written descriptions or polices related to the organization's defined ethics mechanism(s), such as the process for accessing a consultation from the ethics committee;

- written minutes or summaries from the ethics committee's meetings or case consultations;

- written codes of ethics, including the organization's conflict-of-interest policy for the governing body, managers, and staff;

- the organization's mission and values statements;

- written evidence of staff education related to rights and ethics, such as an educational plan, curriculum, or in-service calendars; and

- patient educational materials related to rights and ethics, such as a patient or resident informational brochure on how to access an ethics consultation or how to register a complaint within the organization.

Figure 4-7	Ethics Committee Self-Assessment Tool
	Midwest Bioethics Center

Prologue

Members of the **Kansas City Regional Ethics Committee Consortium** sponsored by **Midwest Bioethics Center** created an ad hoc task force to develop a Self-Assessment Tool for ethics committees. The impetus for this project was a general concern that to date, members of ethics committees have not spent sufficient time evaluating their own performances or that of the committee. Furthermore, members of ethics committees usually have little if anything to compare with their experience. Therefore, it was believed that the collective experiences and wisdom of the ad hoc task force could serve members of the Consortium and others by creating a tool for evaluating the work of ethics committees.

The ad hoc committee that developed this instrument was composed of people with considerable ethics committee experience. In addition, it was reviewed by persons who, collectively, serve on more than three dozen committees at various stages of development and maturation in a variety of institutions. The purpose of this document is to assist members of ethics committees to evaluate their own progress by comparing it with certain benchmarks that committee members believe indicate quality in the work of an ethics committee. It is anticipated that this instrument will be an educational tool rather than a report card.

It should be noted that assertions made in the response section are generalized from the experiences of ethics committee members and that "there is an exception to every rule." Particular ethics committees may decide differently from members of the task force, and there may be good justifications for doing so.

Instructions

The Self-Assessment Tool should be distributed to committee members, and they should each be asked to complete the instrument and make any notes directly on the document

Members should be directed to bring their completed document to the next meeting and be prepared to discuss their responses.

The Response Sheet should be distributed at a regular ethics committee meeting and committee members should collectively review their responses and compare them to those on the companion Response Sheet. (More than one meeting may be required to complete this task.)

Bioethics Development Group

In 1993 **Midwest Bioethics Center** created a separate division known as **Bioethics Development Group** to consult with health care providing organizations throughout the United States on the development, education and maintenance of quality ethics committees. For more information on this survey or consulting services please call or write the address on the cover.

Section I. Inner Workings of the Committee

1. Is your committee multidisciplinary? Do people representing the following disciplines or perspectives serve on your ethics committee?
- ❑ Physician
- ❑ Community representative
- ❑ Nurse
- ❑ Philosopher/person with ethics education
- ❑ Social worker
- ❑ Administrative liaison
- ❑ Chaplain/clergy

2. How many people serve on your ethics committee?
- ❑ Fewer than 7
- ❑ 8 to 15
- ❑ More than 15

(continued)

Figure 4-7	Ethics Committee Self-Assessment Tool
(continued)	Midwest Bioethics Center

3. Do members of our committee serve specified terms? If so, how long are the terms?
   ❑ Yes   ❑ No
   ❑ If yes, 1 year   ❑ If yes, 2 years   ❑ If yes, 3 years   ❑ If yes, 4 years

4. How often does your committee met?
   ❑ As needed   ❑ Monthly   ❑ Every 6 to 8 weeks   ❑ Quarterly

5. Do ethics committee meetings start and end on time?
   ❑ Yes   ❑ No

6. Does the committee meet at a standing time?
   ❑ Yes   ❑ No

7. Are committee members informed about continuing education opportunities? If yes, what percentage of the committee membership participates in continuing education programs and activities?
   ❑ Yes   ❑ No   ___ % who participate

8. Does your committee have an attendance requirement?
   ❑ Yes   ❑ No

9. Do committee members refer to one another by first names?
   ❑ Yes   ❑ No   ❑ Titles are used for some, but not for others

10. Do all committee members vote?
   ❑ Yes   ❑ No

Section II. Educational Responsibilities (Internal and External)

1. Has your committee done education for its members about the following?
   ❑ Ethics or ethical theory   ❑ History of bioethics
   ❑ Clinical ethics   ❑ Health law
   ❑ Religious and cultural values   ❑ Committee process and interpersonal communications

2. Are members of your committee informed about ethical issues associated with the following?
   ❑ Do-not-resuscitate orders   ❑ Imperiled newborns
   ❑ Advance directives   ❑ Surrogate decision makers
   ❑ Withholding/withdrawing   ❑ Care of persons who are HIV positive
      life sustaining treatment

3. Are members of your committee knowledgeable about the following cases and their reasons for being considered important?
   ❑ Claire Conroy   ❑ Nancy Beth Cruzan
   ❑ Karen Ann Quinlan   ❑ Angela Carder

4. Does your committee have a continuing education plan?
   ❑ Yes   ❑ No

5. Does your committee engage in the following educational activities?
   ❑ New employee orientation
   ❑ CEU approved programs for clinical staff
   ❑ Ethics rounds
   ❑ "Brown bag" lunch case discussions
   ❑ Presentations for medical staff departmental meetings
   ❑ Presentations for the nursing staff, social workers and other allied health professionals
   ❑ Presentations for departmental managers, directors or supervisors
   ❑ Education programs for your board of directors

(continued)

Figure 4-7   **Ethics Committee Self-Assessment Tool**
(continued)   **Midwest Bioethics Center**

6. Does your committee provide information about the committee itself to the following?
   - ❏ Consumers
   - ❏ Clinicians
   - ❏ Professional students
   - ❏ Residents
   - ❏ Family members
   - ❏ Board of Trustees

Section III. Case Review

1. Who may ask for a case to be reviewed by the ethics committee?
   - ❏ Patient
   - ❏ Patient's family and other surrogates
   - ❏ Attending physician
   - ❏ Consulting physicians
   - ❏ Nursing staff
   - ❏ Social worker
   - ❏ Chaplain
   - ❏ Patient representative

2. Does your committee engage in expedited review?
   If so, how quickly can the committee or a subcommittee be convened to review a case?
   ❏ Yes   ❏ No   ❏ If yes, within 24 hours   ❏ If yes, within 48 hours
   ❏ If yes, other, explain:_____

3. Before a case review, which of the following are required?
   - ❏ Interview with person requesting consultation
   - ❏ Interview with attending physician
   - ❏ Interview with patient or with appropriate surrogate
   - ❏ Interview with nurse responsible for coordinating care plan
   - ❏ Review of chart

4. Does your committee have written procedures for doing a case consultation?
   ❏ Yes   ❏ No

5. How are consultations reported and to whom?
   - ❏ Verbally
   - ❏ Written in the patient's medical chart
   - ❏ Written by the chair or a designated committee member
   - ❏ Recorded on a special form
   - ❏ Reported to the person requesting the consultation
   - ❏ Reported to the attending physician
   - ❏ Reported to all persons who participate in the consultation
   - ❏ Reported to the full committee (when consultation is done by teams or sub-committees)

Section IV. Policy Development

1. Does your ethics committee's policy include the following?
   - ❏ Mission statement or charge
   - ❏ Description of functions
   - ❏ Statement of jurisdiction, that is, is the committee accountable to administration, the medical staff or the board of directors
   - ❏ Description of membership and terms
   - ❏ Description of how the chair is selected and terms of office
   - ❏ Description of case review process

2. Has your committee reviewed or assisted in developing policies about the following issues?
   - ❏ Do-not-resuscitate orders
   - ❏ Do-not-resuscitate orders for patients undergoing surgery or invasive procedures
   - ❏ Advance directives and the requirements of the Patient Self-Determination Act
   - ❏ Withholding/withdrawing life-sustaining treatment
   - ❏ Care of persons with infectious diseases (including HIV)
   - ❏ Brain death

(continued)

Figure 4-7	Ethics Committee Self-Assessment Tool
(continued)	Midwest Bioethics Center

❏ Surrogate decision makers
❏ Informed consent
❏ Role of minors in treatment decision making
❏ Utilization of intensive care units

3. How often are policies reviewed by the committee?
   ❏ As needed   ❏ Annually   ❏ Bi-annually

4. Does the committee have procedures for becoming involved in policy development/review? Do these procedures answer the following questions?
   ❏ Does the committee need approval before developing policy on its own?
   ❏ Who can request policy review/development?
   ❏ To whom does the committee report policy work?

This tool can be used in assessing the effectiveness of your organization's ethics committee function. CEU, continuing education unit.

Source: Midwest Bioethics Center, Kansas City, Missouri. Used with permission.

Leadership and Staff Interviews

To assess how well the organization implements its rights and ethics policies and mechanisms, the surveyors interview both leaders and staff. Among the individuals who are likely to be interviewed are senior leaders; members of the ethics committee or ethics consultation service, if applicable; a patient representative, ombudsman, or advocate; patient or resident care staff, including physicians, nurses, social workers, chaplains, counselors, nursing assistants, therapists; and staff in other departments such as admitting, finance and billing, or customer service. These questions might be conducted as a component of a leadership or multidisciplinary staff interview or during another survey activity such as visits to individual departments, patient or resident care units, or home visits. The surveyors will focus on major areas such as

■ the processes or mechanisms the organization uses to address ethical issues, including any models for decision making;

■ the methods used for involving patients or residents and their families in ethical decision making;

■ staff knowledge of the organization's policies and procedures related to rights and ethics; and

■ the methods used by the organization to measure, assess, and improve its processes related to ethics.

The following sample questions identify in general terms the issues that may be addressed by surveyors during this activity. Specific questions are often suggested by documents or policies that surveyors read during the document review or by observations of patient or resident care or other interviews. Many of the questions will be open ended to encourage participation among the interview participants. Examples of questions that may be asked of staff and leaders, appropriate to their job and scope of responsibility, include the following:

■ What mechanism do you have to address ethical issues that arise in patient or resident care?

■ How do staff, patients or residents, and families access this mechanism?

■ Can you provide an example of how this mechanism was used recently to address an ethical concern?

■ Can you provide examples of the types of ethical concerns that you face in caring for patients or residents?

■ What makes an issue an "ethical" one to you?

■ What structures or processes does the organization have to address patient or resident rights?

■ Can you share several examples of patient or resident rights that your organization supports? How are you involved in implementing any processes that support patient rights?

■ How do you ensure that a patient's or resident's family participates in care decisions, when appropriate?

■ Can you describe the organization's mechanism for responding to a patient or resident complaint or grievance? What is your role in the complaint handling process?

■ What are the components of the organization's code of ethical behavior as it relates to business activities such as marketing and billing? What is your role, if any, in ensuring that the organization implements its code of ethical business behavior?

■ Can you describe the organization's conflict-of-interest policy as it applies to you? Can you provide an example of a situation that might constitute a conflict of interest?

■ How do you protect patient or resident confidentiality?

■ How are patient or resident rights, dignity, and well-being protected during any restraint and seclusion use?

■ What processes does the organization use to address the care of dying patients or residents?

■ How does the organization respect patient or resident religious, spiritual, or cultural beliefs? How is pastoral counseling provided to patients or residents who request such services?

■ How does the organization address any special communication needs of patients or residents (for example, patients or residents who are deaf, blind, illiterate, or unable to communicate verbally)?

■ How are patients and residents advised of their right to formulate an advance directive? If a patient or resident formulates an advance directive, what is your responsibility in honoring it? How is this information documented and communicated?

- How is the integrity of clinical decision making protected despite any internal or external financial incentives?

- How is the process of informed consent addressed (for example, for invasive procedures)?

- What role do you play, if any, in ensuring that patients and residents have access to protective services if necessary? How would you identify a patient or resident as a potential victim of abuse or neglect?

- What role do you play, if any, in implementing the organization's policies and procedures for organ donation and procurement?

- What education have you received on ethical decision making and patient or resident rights?

- How does the organization measure, assess, and improve its mechanisms for addressing patient or resident rights and ethics? Can you provide any examples of how the organization has improved its care or services in the area of rights and ethics?

Patient Interviews

In addition to staff interviews, surveyors may ask patients and their families questions about the organization's processes for addressing rights and ethics. These interviews often occur during the tour of the patient or resident care units or during home visits to individual patient residences. The focus of the questions is often determined by other observations that the surveyors may have made during the document review and leadership and staff interviews. The following list provides examples of the types of questions that patients or residents may be asked related to this function:

- Were you provided with a copy of your rights as a patient or resident when you were admitted to this health care organization?

- Were you informed about your right to formulate an advance directive (as applicable to those organizations that are required by law and regulation to provide this information to patients or residents upon admission)?

- Are you familiar with the organization's process for registering a complaint or grievance? Have you ever had to use this process? If so, did you find it to be an effective one?

- How well do you feel that the organization has respected your rights as a patient or resident in areas such as privacy or confidentiality?

- How has the organization involved you and your family in decision making about your care?

- If you signed a consent for an invasive procedure such as surgery or endoscopy, how was this consent obtained? How were the risks and benefits of the procedure explained to you and by whom?

- Have you been provided with information about any financial and other responsibilities that you may have for your care?

Implementing an Ethics Mechanism

Implementing effective rights and ethics mechanisms is no easy task in any health care organization. Its impact stretches across all activities of the organization, from the admission function to patient care activities to management decision making and marketing and billing practices. As noted throughout this book, the rights and ethics function is simply too interwoven into the fabric of organization life to confine it strictly to the activities accomplished by one committee or by the management group. Although leadership commitment is essential, organization structures such as policies, procedures, rights and responsibilities documents, mission and values statements, and codes of ethics can provide a useful foundation for implementing these processes in daily life. Staff education and ethics awareness exercises can also be useful in creating a climate where ethical thinking is part of everyday decision making. In the following chapter, sample case scenarios are presented that organizations can use or adapt for staff training and discussion. Additional educational tools are listed in the Resources on page 129.

References

1. Hoffman D, Boyle P, Levenson S: *Handbook for Nursing Home Ethics Committees.* Washington, DC: American Association of Homes and Services for the Aging, 1995.

2. Personal communication. Kathy Freilinger, RN, Iowa Lutheran Hospital Bioethics Committee, Des Moines, IA.

3. Thornton BC, Callahan D, Nelson JL: Bioethics education: Expanding the circle of participants. *Hastings Cent Rep* 23(1):25-29, 1993.

4. Personal communication. Camille Renella, RN, Clinical Medical Ethicist and Associate Faculty, MacLean Center for Clinical Medical Ethics, University of Chicago.

5. Personal communication. David Ozar, PhD, Director, Loyola University of Chicago Center for Ethics.

6. Personal communication. Rev. Julie Ruth Harley, Vice President of Ministry and Mission, Lifelink Corporation, Bensenville, IL.

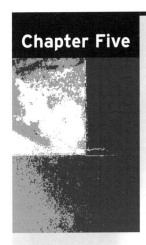

Chapter Five

Case Study Examples and Discussion Questions

The case study approach to ethical analysis is one of the most effective ways of integrating theoretical concepts with practical examples of patient clinical cases or organization situations that occur in most health care organizations on a regular basis. For example, the case of Mr Brown, the terminally ill patient who was requesting cardiopulmonary resuscitation (CPR) in Chapter 1, raised numerous questions about individual autonomy versus the common good, the physician's duties of beneficence and nonmaleficence, distributive justice, the patient's life story or narrative, and personal and spiritual values. Although no clear-cut answers were decided upon, the case of Mr Brown was analyzed through the lens of a variety of ethical approaches or theories as well as through a practical framework for reflection, which is summarized in Table 5-1 (page 122) and discussed fully in Chapter 1 (beginning on page 14).

The hypothetical case study examples and discussion questions that follow are intended to be used as a basis for staff discussion and education in a variety of health care settings, especially in those organizations that are just beginning to formalize their processes for ethical analysis. Refer to the discussions of Mr Brown's case throughout Chapter 1 in regard to various ethical approaches as you answer the discussion questions following each case. Many of the materials listed in the Resources section on page 129 provide additional sources of case studies as well as extensive commentary on current issues in bioethics.

Case Study 1: The Case of Adam

Adam is a 40-year-old man with acquired immunodeficiency syndrome (AIDS) who was referred for home infusion therapy following hospitalization for an opportunistic respiratory infection. He is homosexual and lives alone in a well-maintained townhome. Adam has not revealed his sexual orientation or diagnosis to any of his family members, including his parents and his sister Mary, all of whom live more than 2,000 miles away. To help him with his home antibiotic therapy until he can manage independently, Mary offers to move in with Adam for the first week he is at home. Because she has difficulty arranging for child care for her toddler, Mary decides to bring her daughter Jessica along on the trip. Jessica is rambunctious and inquisitive, and she likes to explore her surroundings.

During the admission visit, the home health nurse examines Adam. He reveals privately that he has not told his family his diagnosis and does not intend to if he can avoid it. He shares, "I'm dealing with more than I can handle right now. I don't need their judgments on top if it." When the nurse asks about his sister, Adam states, "I'll see how it goes. Mary and I have always had a pretty good relationship, even if we don't see each other that often. She only knows that I've had pneumonia." When the nurse inquires about whether he has an advance directive, Adam becomes quiet and then says, "I suppose I should think about it, but to me that means giving up. I'm not ready to do that yet." He agrees to read the written information that the nurse has included in his admission packet.

On the nurse's third visit a few days later, Mary walks her out to the car and in a worried voice says, " He just doesn't seem to be getting any stronger, and he has no appetite. Do you think that there might be more going on here than what we've

Table 5-1	
Framework for Ethical Inquiry	

- Gather and analyze the facts;

- Reflect on the values, principles, and duties involved;

- Explore possible choices; and

- Determine the best possible solution.

been told?" The nurse feels uncomfortable with her questions, but answers that sometimes it takes awhile for the drug treatment to work.

Adam completes his course of antibiotic therapy and Mary returns to her home. His condition continues to deteriorate over the next several weeks and his physician orders a narcotic for severe peripheral neuropathy. During one visit, he asks the home health nurse, "I'm just curious...how much of this stuff would it take to overdose? My doctor told me to take as much as I need."

Discussion Questions

1. What are the facts in this case?

2. What ethical values, principles, and duties are involved?

3. How might you analyze this case using various ethical approaches or perspectives, such as consequentialism, nonconsequentialism, positivism, narrative ethics, or ethics of care?

4. Does the presence of a vulnerable child in the home make any difference to the ethical questions involved? Why or why not?

5. Are there any legal standards that should be considered in Adam's case?

6. How might narrative ethics, or knowing Adam's "story," inform his caregivers?

7. How should the home health nurse proceed with Adam's care?

Case Study 2: The Case of Mrs B

Mrs B is a 72-year-old widow with severe Parkinson's disease who is no longer able to live at home independently because of her ataxia, frequent falls, and difficulties managing the activities of daily living. She lives on a limited income and cannot afford to hire an around-the-clock caregiver so that she will be able to remain at home. Her closest relative, a nephew, lives in another state and has not seen her in many months. Several weeks ago Mrs B was admitted to a long term care facility after a fall at home which resulted in a fractured hip. She recently put her home, where she lived with her husband for 45 years until his death last year, up for sale.

During her nursing home stay, Mrs B becomes increasingly withdrawn and is frequently found sleeping in bed. She refuses her physical therapy treatments, complaining of pain, and says to one of the nursing assistants, "Why bother? I'll just fall again anyway." Mrs B's roommate, who has mild dementia, was found rummaging through Mrs B's clothing drawer by the evening shift nursing assistant. Later, Mrs B angrily tells the assistant, "This isn't like home. Look at this . . . . You can't have any privacy and people are always after me to do things I don't want to do, like walk! It's more like a prison."

The next day, Mrs B asks to speak with the nursing home social worker to inform her of an intent to return home. The social worker tries to explore the possibility of arranging for assistance for Mrs B, such as an attendant or home-delivered meals, but Mrs B refuses all the alternatives presented. " I don't care if you think I'm not safe. I'd rather just go home and die in my own surroundings. What's there to live for, anyway?"

Discussion Questions

1. What are the facts in Mrs B's case?

2. What ethical values, principles, and duties are involved?

3. How might you analyze this case using various ethical approaches or perspectives, such as consequentialism, nonconsequentialism, positivism, narrative ethics, or ethics of care?

4. Does Mrs B have a right to refuse her physical therapy? What if she develops immobility-associated complications, such as a pressure ulcer?

5. What options might the staff pursue in further exploring and treating Mrs B's apparent depression? Does her depression change any of the variables in the case?

6. What alternatives might the nursing home staff explore in Mrs B's care? How should her family be included in the decision making about her care?

Case Study 3: The Case of Baby C and Sylvia

Baby C, now three weeks old, was born at University Hospitals at 30 weeks' gestation. She weighed 3 pounds 12 ounces. Her mother, Sylvia, is a 19-year-old college freshman who received essentially no prenatal care, primarily because of her psychological denial about her pregnancy. Even Sylvia's roommate was unaware of her pregnancy until she developed severe abdominal pain in her dorm room and, as a result, sought medical treatment. While home from college at spring break, Sylvia wore baggy sweatshirts to camouflage her 12-pound weight gain, which she attributed to stress and overeating while studying for final exams. Baby C's father, a student at another university, was someone Sylvia met at a party after she had been drinking heavily one weekend. She has had no contact with him since that night.

Baby C was born with several physical problems, including respiratory distress syndrome and some apparently mild neurological problems. During her three-week stay in the neonatal intensive care unit (NICU), she has received treatment for pneumonia and hyperbilirubinemia. Her condition now seems to be improving steadily and she has been gaining weight. Sylvia visits Baby C in the hospital every afternoon for 30 minutes before she goes to her job as a supermarket cashier. She appears caring and concerned about her baby, yet the NICU nurses also view her as immature for her age and naive about her responsibilities as a mother.

During one late afternoon hospital visit, Sylvia approaches the medical resident to ask when Baby C will be ready for discharge, telling her, "I've found a little apartment near campus that I'm moving into next week. If I cut my classes down to only two a semester, I think I should be able to handle a baby and school too." When the resident asks Sylvia about what kind of support system she has, Sylvia admits that she hasn't told her parents, with whom she has an emotionally distant relationship, about the birth of Baby C. "I guess it's just the two of us now." Sylvia is quiet and vague when the social worker is asked to see her about future discharge plans and follow-up at home. At the unit case rounds the next day, several of the nursing staff express their concerns about Sylvia's ability to care for her infant at home. One of the nurses states, "I know we can arrange for a public health nurse follow-up at home, but is that enough? I just don't think it's ethical to send a newborn home with a mother we're not sure we can trust. It just doesn't feel right."

Discussion Questions

1. What are the facts of the case of Baby C and Sylvia?

2. What ethical values, principles, and duties are involved?

3. How might you analyze this case using various ethical approaches or perspectives, such as consequentialism, nonconsequentialism, positivism, narrative ethics, or ethics of care?

4. What legal standards, if any, are appropriate to consider?

5. What further information would be helpful to know about Sylvia and Baby C before making a recommendation on any ethical issues involved in this case?

6. How should the NICU staff, including the resident, proceed in this case?

Case Study 4: The Case of Mr D

Mr D is the vice president of operations for a 500-bed suburban hospital. His management responsibilities encompass eight hospital departments, including information management. The hospital is undertaking a major enhancement of its computer system, and Mr D is the senior management representative on the task force overseeing its implementation. Three computer vendors are bidding on the multimillion dollar project, and a decision on the choice of vendor will be made within the next several weeks.

A representative of one of the bidding vendor organizations meets Mr D for lunch at a lovely restaurant. None of the other task force members is invited to the lunch meeting, nor are they aware of it. At the meeting, the vendor representative suggests that Mr D attend, all expenses paid, an upcoming weekend seminar that the firm is hosting for its user clients in Palm Springs. "You can talk to some of our users and get in a few rounds of golf at the same time. It's a great way to kill two birds with one trip."

Mr D thinks about the invitation for a few days, then decides to accept. He tells his wife, "After all, they make millions of dollars off hospitals like ours. A few of us folks in the trenches might as well take a little of it back. If anyone deserves a reward for the long hours I've been putting in on this project, it's me. Anyway, it's a drop in the bucket to them. Besides, it might be helpful to talk with some other users before we decide which vendor to use."

Discussion Questions

1. What are the facts in this case?

2. Is there an ethical conflict inherent in this case? Why or why not?

3. How might you analyze this case using various ethical approaches or perspectives, such as consequentialism, nonconsequentialism, or positivism?

4. How should Mr D have handled this situation?

5. What organization "checks and balances" would help to avoid situations like this one from occurring?

Case Study 5: The Case of Eva

Eva is a 35-year-old woman who was diagnosed with metastatic breast cancer two years ago. She lives with her husband and their two small children at home. Until a recent hospitalization for severe pain in her hip and sacral spine, she has been getting along fairly comfortably at home and has been ambulatory. However, she has had continued problems with chronic diarrhea and some muscle wasting, which her physician believes to be due to the side effects of the chemotherapy as well as to her disease progression. While in the hospital, she had a central venous catheter inserted to receive total parenteral nutrition. Eva has gained five pounds in the past week and feels as though she has a great deal more energy.

During this hospitalization, the physician also finds that Eva has a tumor pressing on her spinal cord and recommends radiation therapy. Her physician discusses the treatment alternatives openly with Eva and her husband and recommends that chemotherapy be discontinued. He also suggests that they consider a referral to the local hospice program, stating, "I think you could really use the support for both of you and your children. Hospice helps patients like you who are having problems with pain management." He tells them that Eva's likely prognosis is a matter of several months.

Eva and her husband discuss the possible alternatives and decide that they prefer that she return home with the children as soon as possible and continue to receive outpatient radiation therapy for the next few weeks. Because she feels so much stronger since beginning the total parenteral nutrition, Eva would like it to be continued at home as well, thinking, "Maybe it will give me a little more quality time with my kids." Finally, because they know Eva's likely survival time is limited, they are interested in exploring hospice care and ask that the hospital social worker arrange for a referral.

The liaison nurse from hospice schedules an appointment to meet with Eva, her husband, and the social worker at the hospital. At the planning meeting, the social worker shares that she has checked Eva's insurance coverage and discovered that it includes a hospice benefit that will pay the hospice program $100 per day for "all palliative services provided under the hospice plan of care," including home nursing care, counseling, home health aide services, medications, and equipment such as a hospital bed and an infusion pump. Upon hearing this, the hospice liaison nurse notes that hospice benefit care doesn't usually include radiation therapy or parenteral nutrition. Eva's husband says in a concerned voice, "I don't understand why it wouldn't be covered. The doctor says the radiation will help her pain and hopefully prevent her from becoming paralyzed. After all, I thought that hospice was about quality of life. That's what your brochure says."

Discussion Questions

1. What are the relevant facts?

2. Is Eva an appropriate candidate for hospice care? Why or why not?

3. What are the ethical principles, values, and duties in this case?

4. How might you analyze this case using various ethical approaches or perspectives, such as consequentialism, nonconsequentialism, positivism, narrative ethics, or ethics of care?

5. Is it ethical for the hospice program to limit Eva's treatment options due to concerns about inadequate reimbursement for these services from her insurance company?

6. How should *palliative care* be defined?

7. How should *quality of life* be defined?

8. How should the hospice program describe its philosophy and scope of services in its informational brochure?

Case Study 6: The Case of Mr F

Mr F is a 45-year-old engineer who suffered a traumatic brain injury in a motor vehicle accident while on his way to his work one morning. He is hospitalized at a tertiary medical center in his community on the critical care unit. Mr F's cardiac and respiratory functions are being supported by medications and mechanical ventilation, and his brain activity appears minimal. His physicians believe that his prognosis is very poor and have communicated this information to his family, including his wife, their two teenage children, and his parents. Mr F had not formulated an advance directive.

At a family conference, Mr F's primary physician discusses his prognosis as well as possible alternatives for his treatment. Discontinuation of the ventilator and possible organ donation are raised as possibilities. However, his family is not yet ready to consider such alternatives. His father says to the physician, "How can you even suggest that possibility after only 5 days! He's a young man with a family after all—who knows how he might bounce back? You people wait around like vultures for the next kidney or liver! This is my son you're talking about and we want everything done!" His wife is still in a state of shock over the accident and responds only by saying, "This is more than I can handle right now. I could never forgive myself for killing him if we removed his ventilator. It would be against my religion."

After another week on the critical care unit, Mr F's condition appears unchanged, and his family has not changed their view that they "want everything done" for him. Because of his extensive physical-care needs, Mr F cannot be transferred to a general medical-surgical unit within the hospital. One day the utilization review manager at the hospital approaches Mr F's physician about the long-term plan for this patient, noting, "He's got good insurance coverage, but

I think we need to be proactive here. The coverage won't keep up indefinitely. We need to get the family to be more realistic about his prognosis and treatment."

The physician later states to one of his colleagues, "I can't win. The family won't let me give up on him, and utilization review at the hospital wants me to push on them more to get him out of the critical care unit. On top of all that, the transplant team checks in with me every day just to get an update. I feel like I'm the 'bad guy' in all this and don't know what else to do." His colleague suggests a referral to the ethics consultation team.

Discussion Questions

1. What are the facts of the case of Mr F?
2. What ethical values, principles, and duties are involved?
3. How might you analyze this case using various ethical approaches or perspectives, such as consequentialism, nonconsequentialism, positivism, narrative ethics, or ethics of care?
4. What legal standards, if any, are appropriate to consider?
5. Assuming that you are a member of the ethics consultation team, how might you gather more information about the case in order to make an informed recommendation? Who should be included in the decision-making process?
6. How should Mrs F's religious beliefs be respected in the decisions about her husband's care?
7. How should the organization balance the clinical care and decision making for Mr F against the financial concerns of the organization? Should the utilization review manager be involved in any ethics discussions with the physician and family?
8. What recommendations do you have for the role of the transplant team in the decision making about Mr F's medical treatment?

Case Study 7: The Case of Gina

Gina is a 10-year-old girl whose parents emigrated to the United States from southeast Asia several years ago. Recently, her teacher noticed that Gina was becoming somewhat clumsy at school, and the other children began teasing her after she fell down on the playground several times. The teacher had her evaluated by the school nurse, who detected some subtle neurological changes and recommended that Gina's parents seek a further medical evaluation. Gina is hospitalized for a medical workup and a computed tomography (CT) scan of her brain reveals that Gina has a life-threatening tumor requiring immediate surgery.

With the help of an interpreter, the neurosurgeon discusses this urgent need with Gina's parents and attempts to obtain their consent. They refuse, however, basing their judgment on their deeply held cultural and religious beliefs that a person's spirit resides within the skull. Opening the skull through an invasive procedure such as surgery might release that spirit and the essence of the person. Although they understand the seriousness of the tumor and its potential impact, they will not give their consent for the neurosurgery. The physician is angry and frustrated with this choice, and consults the hospital's chaplain, who is also a member of the ethics committee, stating, "I know we need to be sensitive to the parents' religious beliefs, but how can that be important enough to risk the life of a child? Isn't there some other approach?" The chaplain suggests an immediate ad hoc meeting of the entire ethics committee to discuss this case and provide recommendations to the physician and parents.

Discussion Questions

1. What are the facts in Gina's case?

2. What ethical values, principles, and duties are involved?

3. How might you analyze this case using various ethical approaches or perspectives, such as consequentialism, nonconsequentialism, positivism, narrative ethics, or ethics of care?

4. What legal standards, if any, are appropriate to consider? What difference, if any, does it make that this case involves a minor?

5. Assuming that you are a member of the ethics committee how might you gather more information about the case in order to make an informed recommendation? Who might you include in the discussions?

6. To what extent should health care professionals and organizations respect the religious, spiritual, and cultural beliefs of patients and families in recommending medical treatments?

Incorporating Ethics into Everyday Practice

As stated many times throughout this book, the study of ethics in health care is by nature without absolutes. Even among colleagues of integrity who are well-versed in ethical theory, principles, and values, it may be difficult to achieve a consensus about what is "right" or "wrong" in an ethically complex situation. In these situations as well as through case study examples, a thoughtful analysis of the facts, values, and possible theoretical approaches can help to inform our thinking about how to approach this decision making, even if it seems that in the process we open more avenues of inquiry, potential confusion, and frustration. The more we understand about our individual values and beliefs as well as about ethical theories, legal precedents, and our own organization policies, the greater the chance that the conclusions reached will have a measure of internal consistency, logical validity, and supportability.

But getting to this point is often a challenge—the challenge of "muddling through" what can sometimes seem like a mind-boggling maze of approaches and considerations. However, by designing a thoughtful framework to address both clinical and organization ethical issues—including written policies and procedures, patient or resident rights documents, staff educational resources, and mechanisms such as ethics committees, interdisciplinary teams, and ethics consultants for responding to ethical concerns—today's health care organization can successfully equip itself to respond to the challenge of incorporating ethical thinking into its daily practices.

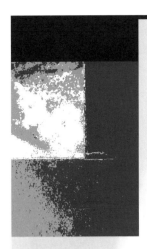

Resources

The following is a listing of available resources related to patient rights and ethics that a health care organization may want to use in developing educational materials for ethics committees, ethics consultation teams, and leadership and staff training. It includes

- journals and newsletters (page 131),
- books and pamphlets (page 131),
- ethics resources on the Internet (page 133),
- ethics resource centers (page 134), and
- professional societies and associations (page 135).

This listing is not intended to be an exhaustive directory of all available resources, yet it provides a useful direction in developing or enhancing a bioethics library.

Journals and Newsletters

*The American Journal of Law
and Medicine*
765 Commonwealth Avenue
Boston, MA 02215

Bioethics
Blackwell Publishing
238 Main Street, Suite 501
Cambridge, MA 02142

Bioethics Examiner
Center for Bioethics
University of Minnesota
Suite N504
410 Church Street
Minneapolis, MN 55455-0346

Bioethics Forum
Midwest Bioethics Center
1021-1025 Jefferson Street
Kansas City, MO 64105-1329

*Cambridge Quarterly of Health
Care Ethics*
Cambridge University Press
40 W 20th Street
New York, NY 10011-4211

Communique
Center for Ethics and Human Rights
American Nurses Association
600 Maryland Avenue, SW
Suite 100 West
Washington, DC 20024-2571

Hastings Center Report
The Hastings Center
255 Elm Road
Briarcliff Manor, New York 10510

The Hospice Journal
The Hayworth Press, Inc
10 Alice Street
Binghamton, NY 13904-1580

Kennedy Institute of Ethics Resources
Johns Hopkins University Press
2715 N Charles Street
Baltimore, MD 21218

Journal of Clinical Ethics
University Publishing Group, Inc
107 E Church Street
Frederick, MD 21701

Journal of Law, Medicine, and Ethics
765 Commonwealth Avenue
Boston, MA 02215

Journal of Medicine and Philosophy
Kluwer Academic Publishing
PO Box 358, Accord Station
Hingham, MA 02018

Medical Ethics Advisor
American Health Consultants
PO Box 740056
Atlanta, GA 30374

Medical Humanities Review
Institute for the Medical Humanities
The University of Texas Medical Branch
Galveston, TX 77555-1311

Books and Pamphlets

Autonomy and Long Term Care
George J Agich
New York: Oxford University Press, 1993

*Choices and Conflict: Explorations in
Health Care Ethics*
Emily Friedman (ed)
Chicago: American Hospital Publishing,
1992

*Classic Cases in Medical Ethics:
Accounts of Cases That Have Shaped
Medical Ethics, with Philosophical,
Legal, and Historical Backgrounds,
2nd edition*
Gregory E Pence (ed)
New York: McGraw Hill, 1995

Books and Pamphlets (continued)

Code of Medical Ethics: Current Opinions with Annotations
American Medical Association Council on Ethical and Judicial Affairs
Chicago: American Medical Association, 1996

Contemporary Issues in Bioethics, 4th edition
Tom L Beauchamp and LeRoy Walters (eds)
Belmont, CA: Wadsworth Publishing, 1994

Ethical and Legal Issues in Home Health and Long-Term Care: Challenges and Solutions
Dennis A Robbins
Gaithersburg, MD: Aspen Publishers, 1996

Ethical Dimensions of Pharmaceutical Care
Amy M Haddad and Robert A Buerki (eds)
New York: Hayworth Press, 1996

Ethical Issues in Death and Dying, 2nd edition
Tom L Beauchamp and Robert M Veatch (eds)
Englewood Cliffs, NJ: Prentice Hall, 1995

Ethics Committees: Allies in Long Term Care
American Association of Homes and Services (AAHS) for the Aging and the American Association of Retired Persons (AARP)
Washington, DC: AAHS and AARP, 1990

Ethics for Everyone: A Practical Guide to Interdisciplinary Biomedical Ethics Education
Linda C Grafius
Chicago: American Hospital Publishing, 1995

Ethics in an Aging Society
Harry R Moody
Baltimore: Johns Hopkins University Press, 1992

Ethics in Nursing, 3rd edition
Martin Benjamin and Jay Curtis
New York: Oxford University Press, 1992

The Ethics of the Ordinary in Healthcare: Concepts and Cases
John Abbott Worthley
Chicago: Health Administration Press, 1997

The Foundations of Bioethics, 2nd edition
Tristram H Engelhardt, Jr
New York: Oxford University Press, 1996

Health Care Ethics Committees: The Next Generation
Judith W Ross, et al
Chicago: American Hospital Publishing, 1993

Health Care Ethics: Critical Issues for the 21st Century
John F Monagle and David C Thomasma
Frederick, MD: Aspen Publishers, 1997

If I Were a Rich Man Could I Buy a Pancreas? and Other Essays on the Ethics of Health Care (Medical Ethics Series)
Arthur L Caplan
Bloomington, IN: Indiana University Press, 1992

International Directory of Bioethics Organizations
Anita L Nolan and Mary C Coutts (eds)
Washington, DC: Georgetown University Kennedy Institute of Ethics, 1993

Life Choices: A Hastings Center Introduction to Bioethics
Joseph H Howell, William F Sale, and Daniel Callahan (eds)
Washington, DC: Georgetown University Press, 1995

Books and Pamphlets (continued)

The McGraw Hill Guide Pocket Guide to Managed Care: Business, Practice, Law, Ethics
John LaPuma and David Schiedermayer
New York: McGraw Hill, 1996

Medical Ethics, 2nd edition
Robert M Veatch
Boston: Jones and Bartlett Publishers, 1996

Medical Ethics: Policies, Protocols, Guidelines, and Programs
John F Monagle and David C Thomasma (eds)
Gaithersburg, MD: Aspen Publishers
(updated annually)

Moral Matters: Ethical Issues in Medicine and the Life Sciences
Arthur L Caplan
New York: John Wiley and Sons, 1994

Opinions of the Ethics Committee on the Principles of Medical Ethics
American Psychiatric Association
Washington, DC: American Psychiatric Association, 1995

Principles of Biomedical Ethics, 4th edition
Tom L Beauchamp and James F Childress
New York: Oxford University Press 1994

Standard of Care: The Law of American Bioethics
George J Annas
New York: Oxford University Press, 1993

Ethics Resources on the Internet

American Association for Bioethics
http://www.geog.utah.edu/~aab/

American Society for Bioethics and Humanities
http://www.asbh.org

Center for Bioethics/University of Minnesota
http://www.med.umn.edu/bioethics/

Center for Bioethics/Bioethics Internet Project/University of Pennsylvania
http://www.med.upenn.edu/~bioethic/

Center for Health Care Ethics/ St. Joseph Health System
http://www.chce.org/

The Hastings Center
http://www.cpn.org/section/affiliates/ hastings_center.html

The Joseph and Rose Kennedy Institute of Ethics
http://guweb.georgetown.edu/kennedy/

MacLean Center for Clinical Medical Ethics/University of Chicago
http://ccme.mac4.bsd.uchicago.edu/ CCMEHomePage.html

Medical College of Wisconsin
http://www.mcw.edu/bioethics/

Midwest Bioethics Center
http://www.midbio.org/

Institute for Jewish Medical Ethics
http://www.hia.com/hia/medethic/

Pope John Center for the Study of Ethics in Health Care
http://www.pjcenter.org/PJChome.html

Rush University

Ethics Resource Centers

Center for Bioethics
University of Minnesota
Suite N504
410 Church Street
Minneapolis, MN 55455-0346

Center for Bioethics
University of Pennsylvania
3401 Market Street, #320
Philadelphia, PA 19104-3308

Center for Biomedical Ethics
Case Western Reserve University
School of Medicine, Room T402
10900 Euclid Avenue
Cleveland, Ohio 44106-4976

Center for Biomedical Ethics
University of Virginia
Box 348 HSC
Charlottesville, VA 22908

Center for Clinical Bioethics
Georgetown University Medical Center
4000 Reservoir Road NW
Washington, DC 20007

Center for Clinical Ethics
University of Pittsburgh Department
of Medicine
3400 Forbes Avenue, Suite 506
Pittsburgh, PA 15213

Center for Ethics and Human Rights
American Nurses Association
600 Maryland Avenue SW
Washington, DC 20024-2571

Center for Healthcare Ethics
St Joseph Health System
PO Box 14132
Orange, CA 92863-7690

Center for Health Care Ethics
St Louis University Medical Center
1402 S Grand Boulevard
St Louis, MO 63104

Center for Health Ethics and Law
West Virginia University
G-106 HSN
Morgantown, WV 26506

Center for Medical Ethics
and Health Policy
Baylor College of Medicine
One Baylor Plaza
Houston, TX 77030-3498

Center for Study of Bioethics
Medical College of Wisconsin
8701 Watertown Plank Road
Milwaukee, WI 53226

Creighton University Center
for Health Policy and Ethics
California at 24th Street
Omaha, NE 68178

Ethics Outreach Services Project
Center for Ethics
Loyola University of Chicago
6525 N Sheridan Road
Chicago, IL 60626

The Hastings Center
255 Elm Road
Briarcliff Manor, NY 10510

Institute for Jewish Medical Ethics
645 14th Avenue
San Francisco, CA 94118

Institute for the Medical Humanities
The University of Texas Medical Branch
301 University Blvd.
Galveston, TX 77555-0202

The Joseph and Rose Kennedy
Institute of Ethics
Georgetown University
Box 571212
Washington, DC 20057-1212

MacLean Center for Clinical
Medical Ethics
University of Chicago, MC6098
5841 S Maryland
Chicago, IL 60637

Midwest Bioethics Center
1021-1025 Jefferson Street
Kansas City, MO 64105-1329

Ethics Resource Centers (continued)

Pacific Center for Health Policy
and Ethics
University of Southern California
USC Law Center 444
University Park, CA 90089-0071

The Park Ridge Center for the Study
of Health, Faith, and Ethics
211 E Ontario Street, Suite 800
Chicago, IL 60611-3215

Pope John Center for the Study
of Ethics in Health Care
186 Forbes Road
Braintree, MA 02184

The Poynter Center for the Study
of Ethics and American Institutions
Indiana University
410 N Park Avenue
Bloomington, IN 47405

Stanford University Center
for Biomedical Ethics
701 Welch Road, Suite 1105
Palo Alto, CA 94304

Professional Societies and Associations

American Society for Bioethics and
Humanities *(formed by merger of
American Association for Bioethics,
Society for Bioethics Consultation, and
Society for Health and Human Values)*
4700 West Lake
Glenview, IL 60025-1485

American Society of Law, Medicine,
and Ethics
765 Commonwealth Avenue, 16th floor
Boston, MA 02215

Association for Practical and
Professional Ethics
410 North Park Avenue
Bloomington, IN 47405

Bioethics Consultation Group
2322 Sixth Street, Suite 193
Berkeley, CA 94710

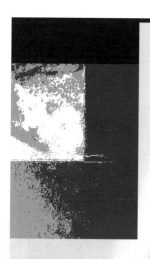

Glossary

advance directive A document or documentation allowing a person to give directions about future medical care or to designate another person(s) to make medical decisions if the patient loses decision-making capacity. Advance directives may include living wills, durable powers of attorney, do-not-resuscitate (DNR) orders, right to die, or similar documents expressing the patient's preferences as specified in the Patient Self-Determination Act.

autonomy The condition of having one's life under one's control and making decisions or plans and acting on them. Autonomy also dictates the duty of individuals not to interfere either intentionally or negligently in another person's making of decisions or plans or acting on them. Autonomy forms the ethical basis for patient's right of autonomy, which includes, among other rights, the right to informed consent, the right to refuse treatment, and the right to die.

beneficence The state or quality of being charitable or producing favorable effects. For example, beneficence towards patients can be defined as preventing harm to them, benefiting them, and, if harm is unavoidable, to make certain the harm is substantially outweighed by the benefit.

bioethics A variously defined term for a multidisciplinary field concerned with the ethical and moral dimensions of the clinical and policy application of research findings in the life sciences and of biomedical research using human subjects. The matter of whether bioethics is a separate discipline as well as the definition of its principles are under debate. "Strangers at the bedside" was the description in the first formal history of the field (1992) to distinguish it from medical ethics. *Clinical ethics* is the term used for bioethics based on real individual cases in the clinical setting. Bioethicists and bioethics centers or commissions draw on traditional ethics, medical ethics, moral philosophy, social science, and theology to confront issues posed by genetic engineering, genetic testing, fetal tissue and embryo research, surrogate reproduction, organ transplantation, abortion, assisted suicide, euthanasia, human experimentation, and other interventions to fulfill the requirements of informed consent. *Synonym:* biomedical ethics.

code of ethics A statement of principles and standards concerning the conduct of those who subscribe to the code, as in a code of ethics that defines proper professional behavior and practices. Codes of ethics are distinguished from licensure laws or practice acts in that they are a form of collective self-regulation rather than of regulation by external bodies.

confidentiality An individual's right, within the law, to personal and informational privacy, including his or her health care records.

conscience clause A law or clause allowing individuals or institutions the right to refuse to perform an activity that is contrary to their moral or religious beliefs.

consequentialism An ethical theory stating that an action is judged in terms of its consequences, that the value of an action is determined by its utility, and that all action should be directed toward achieving the greatest happiness for the greatest number of people. *Synonyms:* axiological ethics; utilitarianism.

Cruzan case (*Cruzan* v *Director, Missouri Dept. of Health,* U.S., 110 S.Ct. 2841 [1990]) This case, involving a young woman left in a persistent vegetative state following an automobile accident, was the first right-to-die case to reach the U.S. Supreme Court. The patient's parents petitioned the court to terminate artificial nutrition and hydration; the patient was not sustained by any life-support machinery. A trial court granted the request; the state supreme court reversed it; and the parents appealed to the U.S. Supreme Court, which upheld the state's requirement of "clear and convincing evidence" that an incompetent patient would wish to have life-sustaining treatment withdrawn before permitting the cessation of such treatment. Additional testimony was supplied to the trial court, which then granted authorization to terminate artificial nutrition and hydration.

decisional capacity The capacity of an individual to understand the ramifications of a decision that must be made, consider the benefits and burdens of various choices, and communicate his or her choices either verbally or nonverbally. In general, individuals with decisional capacity are regarded as capable of providing informed consent to medical treatment.

DNR (do-not-resuscitate) order An order placed in a patient's medical record by an attending physician, with patient or surrogate consent, that directs hospital personnel not to revive the patient if cardiopulmonary arrest occurs. The decision is based on the patient's overall condition and values.

durable power of attorney for health care An advance directive wider in scope than a living will which designates a family member or friend to make decisions about a patient's care should the patient become unable to do so. This type of power of attorney, in contrast to ordinary power of attorney, remains or becomes effective when the principal becomes incompetent to act for herself or himself. *Synonym:* health care proxy.

ethics The branch of philosophy that deals with systematic approaches to moral issues, such as the distinction between right and wrong and the moral consequences of human actions. Ethics involves a system of behaviors, expectations, and morals composing standards of conduct for a population or a profession.

ethics committee A multidisciplinary committee of a health care organization that provides case consultation designed to help resolve moral conflicts that arise in difficult medical cases; educates institutional personnel in the ways in which ethics affects their job responsibilities; and develops institutional policies on various ethical issues.

extraordinary care 1. Use of advanced technology in medical treatment to keep a patient alive, for example, mechanical ventilation. **2.** Care that involves life-supporting medical interventions that offer no significant health improvement or that cannot be administered without excessive pain.

futile care According to the American Medical Association *Code of Medical Ethics* (1994), care that in the physician's judgment will not have a reasonable chance of benefiting the patient. The code asserts that physicians are not ethically obligated to deliver such care and should not provide treatment simply because patients demand it.

futility The absence of a useful purpose or useful result in a diagnostic procedure or therapeutic intervention, in a situation in which a patient's condition will not be improved by treatment or in which treatment preserves permanent unconsciousness or cannot end dependence on intensive medical care. The concept is controversial and, according to the American Medical Association *Code of Medical Ethics* (1994), should not be used to justify denial of treatment because it cannot be meaningfully defined. *Synonym:* medical futility; medically futile.

informed consent In law, the principle that a physician has a duty to disclose what a reasonably prudent physician in the medical community, in the exercise of reasonable care, would disclose to his or her patients about whatever risks of injury might be incurred from a proposed course of treatment, testing, or research. A patient, exercising ordinary care for his or her own welfare, and faced with a choice of undergoing the proposed or alternate treatment, testing, or research, or none at all, may then intelligently exercise judgement by reasonably balancing the probable risks against the probable benefits. *Synonym:* patient consent.

institutional review board (IRB) An organizational committee, mandated in 1981 and since governed by the U.S. Department of Health and Human Services, designated to review and approve biomedical research involving humans as subjects. IRBs provide certain protections for human subjects of research and research proposals only if conditions established by federal regulations are met. Example conditions are minimized risks to which subjects are exposed; reasonable risks to subjects in relation to the anticipated benefits, if any; and the informed consent of all participants is sought and appropriately documented.

life-prolonging procedure Any procedure or intervention, such as artificial ventilation, that prolongs the dying process when death will occur within a short time. *Synonym:* death-delaying procedure; death-prolonging procedure.

life-sustaining procedure Any intervention that is judged likely to be effective in prolonging a patient's life or that is being used to sustain a patient's life. In law, a life-sustaining procedure is one that may be suspended on a court order or pursuant to a living will in the case of, for example, a comatose and terminally ill person. Life-sustaining procedures include mechanical or other artificial means to sustain, restore, or supplant some vital function, such as breathing, which serve to prolong the moment of death when, in the judgment of attending and consulting physicians (as reflected in the patient's medical records), death is imminent if such procedures are not used.

living will Instructional directives in written form that indicate the author's wishes for medical treatment should he or she become incapacitated and unable to participate in medical decision making. Many states have living will legislation, for example, Kansas has the Natural Death Act and Missouri has the Death-Prolonging Procedures Act. *Natural death acts* are pieces of legislation generally enacted to codify living wills and often contain specific examples. *Synonyms:* directive to physicians; medical directive; terminal care document.

medical ethics The principles of proper professional conduct concerning the rights and duties of physicians themselves, their patients, and their fellow practitioners, as well as their actions in the care of patients and in relations with patients' families. In the United States, these principles are embodied in the *Code of Medical Ethics: Current Opinions with Annotations,* maintained and periodically updated by the American Medical Association's Council on Ethical and Judicial Affairs.

nonconsequentialism An ethical theory or system that holds that right or wrong is not determined by assessment of consequences, which distinguishes it from utilitarian ethics. Nonconsequentialism is based on the assumption that value is inherent in the principle or duty. *Synonym:* deontological ethics.

normative ethics Theories that formulate and defend basic moral principles and rules that determine what is right or wrong.

Nuremberg code The set of principles formulated to govern the ethics of research on human beings, following the Nuremberg tribunal at the end of World War II, which declared Nazi physicians guilty of crimes against humanity for experimenting on human beings without their consent. The code forms the underpinnings of the law and ethics of informed consent.

ordinary care Care that will offer reasonable hope of benefit to a patient with less chance of creating the burdens that may be associated with extraordinary care.

organ procurement The process of obtaining vital human organs, such as livers, hearts, and kidneys, for implantation in other humans who need them. Organs can be procured from cadavers or live donors, such as patients on life-support systems who are proclaimed dead.

paternalism A traditional model of the physician-patient relationship in which the physician is held to know what is best for the patient and acts accordingly, sometimes by choosing among alternative treatments without consulting the patient and sometimes by withholding information from the patient, such as the diagnosis of and prognosis for a terminal illness. The concept is under challenge both within and outside the profession with a growing concern for patient autonomy and a growing trend toward patient and family participation and shared decision making.

patient bill of rights A statement of ethical and legal principles adopted by a health care organization to regulate its operational policies and procedures, operations staff, professional staff, and volunteers in a manner that recognizes and obligates the organization to protect and promote the human dignity and rights of patients. *Synonym:* bill of patient rights.

patient participation Patient involvement in the decision-making process in matters pertaining to his or her health.

patient rights Liberties and privileges (for example, autonomy, confidentiality, privacy) that individuals retain during their status as patients, to the extent permitted by law.

Patient Self-Determination Act (PSDA) Legislation passed in the Bush administration (1990) stating that hospitals, skilled nursing facilities, hospices, home health care agencies, and HMOs are responsible for developing patient information for distribution. The information must include patients' rights, advance directives (for example, living wills), ethics committees' consultation and education functions, limited medical treatment (supportive/comfort care only), mental health treatment, resuscitation, restraints, surrogate decision making, and transfer of care. The purpose of the act is to ensure that individuals receiving health care services will be given an opportunity to participate in and direct health care decisions affecting themselves.

Quinlan case [*In re Quinlan,* 70 N.J. 10, 355 A.2d 647 (N.J. 1976) *cert. denied, Garger* v *New Jersey,* 429 U.S. 922 (1976)] A landmark legal case involving Karen Quinlan, a 22-year-old who sustained severe brain damage, became comatose, and remained in a chronic vegetative state. The hospital and physicians refused her parents' request to terminate the mechanical respirator that aided her breathing. The New Jersey Supreme Court approved her father's request to be appointed his daughter's guardian and have the support systems discontinued. The patient continued to breathe on her own, receiving antibiotics and nasogastric tube feedings, until her death in 1985. This decision upheld the doctrine of *substituted judgment* under which an incompetent person's guardian makes a decision that he or she believes reflects the decision the patient would have made had he or she been capable.

resident bill of rights Federal protections for nursing home residents first provided for in OBRA '87 (Omnibus Budget Reconciliation Amendments of 1987). States are also required to have a Bill of Resident Rights which is least as protective as the federal statutes. Provisions outline the minimum standards of respect and caring, privacy, health, safety, patient autonomy, notice requirements, and fiduciary duties of facilities.

restraint Use of a physical, chemical, or mechanical device to involuntarily restrain the movement of the whole or a portion of a patient's body as a means of controlling his or her physical activities to protect him or her or other persons from injury. Restraint differs from mechanisms usually and customarily used during medical, diagnostic, or surgical procedures that are considered a regular part of such procedures. These mechanisms include body restraint during surgery, arm restraint during intravenous administration, and temporary physical restraint before administration of electroconvulsive therapy. Devices used to protect the patient, such as bed rails, tabletop chairs, protective nets, helmets, or the temporary use of halter-type or soft-chest restraints, and mechanisms, such as orthopedic appliances, braces, wheelchairs, or other appliances or devices used to posturally support the patient or assist him or her in obtaining and maintaining normative bodily functions, are not considered restraint interventions.

right of privacy The constitutional right of privacy to prohibit unwanted invasion, especially of one's own body. This right is the basis for informed consent and restriction of governmental intrusion in areas such as birth control, sterilization, abortion, and the right to refuse medical treatment.

right to die The legal right to refuse life-saving or life-sustaining (or death-prolonging) procedures. A competent adult has the legal right to refuse medical treatment, even if that treatment is essential to sustaining life. The question of a patient's right to die arises when a person has a condition that makes his or her quality of life so intolerable that he or she believes that death is preferable. Serious legal and ethical issues arise when the patient is unconscious or incompetent and the decision to withdraw or refuse treatment must be made for him or her by someone else.

Roe* v *Wade [410 U.S. 113 (1973), reh'g denied, 410 U.S. 959 (1973)] The landmark U.S. Supreme Court case that legalized abortion by striking down restrictive state abortion laws as unconstitutional, ruling that those laws violated a woman's right of privacy to make her own decisions concerning her body. The Court held that the state could regulate abortions only where necessary to serve a compelling state interest, defined as protection of the life and health of pregnant women and protecting the "potentiality of human life." The decision did not address, nor did it decide, the question of when life began or when the fetus became a "person."

situation ethics A system of ethics that evaluates acts in light of their situational context rather than by applying moral absolutes.

SUPPORT (Study to Understand Prognoses and Preferences for Outcomes and Risks of Treatment) Prognostic Model A system for making objective estimates of the probable survival of seriously ill, hospitalized adults over a

180-day period, using each patient's diagnosis, age, number of days in the hospital before entry into the study, presence of cancer, neurological function, and 11 physiological variables recorded on day 3 of the study.

Uniform Rights of the Terminally Ill Act A model act designed to provide various means by which a patient's preferences can be carried out with regard to the administration of life-sustaining treatment. The act permits an individual to execute a declaration that instructs a physician to withhold or withdraw life-sustaining treatment in the event the individual is in a terminal condition and is unable to participate in medical treatment decisions or, in the alternative, designates another individual to make decisions regarding the withholding or withdrawal of life-sustaining treatment. Further, the act authorizes an attending physician to withhold or withdraw life-sustaining treatment in the absence of a declaration upon the consent of a close relative if the action would not conflict with the individual's known intentions. A number of states have adopted the act.

vision statement A written description, developed by an organization's leaders, of what the organization wishes to be, what it hopes to achieve, and its relationship to those it serves.

withdrawing treatment Termination or removal of a particular treatment without termination of care. There is no necessary difference (moral or legal) between withdrawing or withholding the same treatment, for example, stopping mechanical ventilation versus not starting mechanical ventilation.

.

Index

A

Advance care planning, 23, 29, 31, 35-36

Advance directives, 5, 24f, 27f, 29, 35, 37f, 40, 56-57f, 102, 108, 110f

  in case study, 8, 15-16, 121, 126

  education about, 8, 29, 36, 41-42f, 48, 59, 60, 95

  and end-of-life care, 29-60

  implementation of, 37-42f, 61f

  right to formulate 5, 23, 29, 34f, 35, 94, 116, 117

  sample policy 43-44, 45-46

  sample questionnaire, 47f

  team, 54, 59-60

Advisory committees. *See* Ethics committees

American College of Healthcare Executives, 72, 82

American Geriatrics Society, 48

American Hospital Association (AHA), 36, 72, 82

  and Patient Bill of Rights, 23, 24-25f, 72

American Medical Association (AMA), 36, 48, 72

  and do-not-resuscitate orders, 12, 13, 17, 36

American Nurses Association (ANA), 36, 48, 72

American Psychiatric Association, 29, 72

American Psychological Association, 29

Americans with Disabilities Act, 27f

Assessment, 4, 59, 83, 93-95, 102-103, 112-115f

  baseline, 94-95, 101

  tool for, 112-115f

Autonomy, 3, 6, 11-12, 67, 96, 121

  and common good, 6, 10, 36

  in geriatrics, 12

  of individuals or patients, 7, 8, 12, 16, 21, 36, 84, 100

  in Kantian theory, 11, 17

  in narrative ethics, 14

  of physicians, 8

B

Behavioral health care organizations, 29, 79, 93, 101

Beneficence, 3, 6, 7, 8, 11-12, 16, 67, 121

Billing, ethics in, 7, 67, 68, 71f, 76, 77, 78f, 87, 108, 115, 116, 118

Bioethics. *See also* Ethics; Organization ethics

  approaches to, 9-14

  definition of, 3, 5-6

  education about, 95-100

  emergence of, 3-5, 96

  and legal precedents, 12-13, 29

  role of, 6

Books, on patient rights and ethics, 131-133

Business ethics. *See* Organization ethics

C

Capacity. *See* Decisional capacity

Cardiopulmonary resuscitation (CPR). *See also* Do-not-resuscitate orders

  appropriate use of, 8, 10, 11-12, 13-14, 16, 35, 36

  and end-of-life care, 35

  physicians' awareness of patients' preferences about, 4, 31

Case studies

  of elderly patient wanting to leave nursing home, 122-123

  of end-of-life decisions, 126-127

and ethical approaches, 7-14

of newborn with young mother,
123-124

of organization ethics, 124-125

of parents who refuse treatment for
child on religious grounds, 127-128

of patient right to confidentiality,
121-122

of terminally ill patient requesting
CPR, 7-14, 15-17, 121

of treatments not covered by
insurance, 125-126

Categorical imperative, 11

Code of ethics, 4, 67, 72, 76-83, 118

and conflicts of interest, 77, 79,
82-83

educating staff to, 94, 95

and Joint Commission, 72-73, 111, 116

organization examples, 77, 78-79f,
80-82f

of professional organizations,
12, 13, 23, 29, 72, 76, 82

Comfort care. See Palliative care

Committees. See Ethics committee

Common good, versus individual,
6, 10, 36

Compassion, 6, 11, 70, 75, 77, 78f

Conduct

codes of ethical, 67, 68, 72, 74f, 76,
82, 84, 93, 95, 98

standards of, 84, 86f, 88-89f, 90f

violations of, 68, 86

Confidentiality, 5, 23, 24f, 26f,
29, 70, 84, 95, 96, 100t, 110f

in case study, 121-122

and Joint Commission standards,
22, 108, 116

Conflicts. See also Grievances

in case study, 124-125

educating staff about, 94, 95

and ethical framework, 15, 93

examples of, 70, 83t, 84t

of interest, 72, 74t, 77, 79,
82-83, 87

and Joint Commission survey
process, 116

policies or statements regarding,
7, 28f, 68, 73, 74t, 76, 84, 111

resolving, 16, 52f

Consent. See Informed consent

Consequentialism, 9-10, 13

Consultation. See Ethics, consultation

Cruzan v Director, Missouri
Department of Health, 12-13, 29, 113f

D

Decisional capacity, 3, 12, 15, 29,
37f, 38f, 43f, 45f, 108, 110f

of minors, 32-35f

and withdrawing life-prolonging
procedures, 50-52f

Deontological ethics, 10, 17

Directives. See Advance directives

Disclosure of information 35, 77, 83

Distributive justice, 5, 8, 16, 100t, 121

Document review, 108, 111

Do-not-resuscitate (DNR) orders, 16,
30f, 31, 38f, 43f, 51f, 55f, 57f, 58f

and American Medical Association,
12, 13, 17

appropriate use of, 35, 36

policy for, 40f

Durable power of attorney for health
care, 24f, 35, 37f, 38f, 42f,
43f, 46f, 63f

E

Education

about advance directives, 41-42f

approaches to, 29, 96-98, 100

brochures, 102, 109f, 110-111f

of community, 36, 41-42f, 59, 60

curriculum for, 95, 96-98, 87t, 99t, 100

designing plan for, 93, 95, 98, 100

by ethics committee, 69, 96, 102, 113-114f

of organization, 7, 95-98, 100, 113-114f

of patients and families, 48, 72, 109f, 111

of physicians, 41f, 48, 60

resources for, 42f, 94, 95, 131-135

of staff, 21, 41f, 54, 59, 60, 68, 76, 83-84, 93, 94-98, 100-102, 111, 117, 118, 121

Educational Development Corporation (EDC), 94-95

End-of-life care, 4, 21, 54, 96, 108

and advance directives, 29, 31, 35-36, 37-42f, 43-44f, 45-46f, 47f, 48, 49-52f, 56-58f

and palliative care, 48, 53-54f, 55f, 58-59f

Equality, 4, 77, 78f

Ethical behavior, 6, 7, 67, 68, 69, 72, 73, 77, 98, 100t, 116

checkpoints for, 71t

Ethical inquiry, 3, 5-6, 7, 101, 109f

model for, 14-17, 121, 122, 128

Ethics. *See also* Bioethics; Organization ethics

assessment of, 94-95

case scenarios, 7, 9-14, 15-17, 48, 60, 121-128

centers for, 134-135

checkpoints for behavior, 71t

and clinical policies and procedures, 21-64, 67

codes of, 4, 7, 12-13, 15, 23, 29, 80-82f, 94, 111, 116, 118

and conflicts, 77, 79, 82-83, 83t, 84t, 127-128,

consultation, 5, 6, 69, 73, 93, 94, 95, 96, 98, 100, 101, 102, 103t, 104f, 105f, 106-108f, 109f, 110-111f, 111, 115, 127, 128

organization examples, 5, 102, 104f, 105f, 106-108f

designing and implementing mechanisms for, 100-102

document checklist, 22

education, 7, 41, 42f, 68, 93, 95-100

curriculum for, 97t, 99t, 100t

monitoring performance of, 83-84, 85f, 86-87, 88-89f, 90f

of organization, 67-90

and organization climate for, 7, 67-70, 76-77, 79, 82-84, 86-87

statement of, 78-79f

Ethics of caring, 13-14

Ethics committee, 4, 93, 97t, 102, 103t, 109-111f, 112-115f, 127, 128

advisory, 7

and consultation, 6, 15, 36, 93, 102, 111

forming, 101, 103

and Institutional Review Board, 4

at Iowa Lutheran Hospital, 95

and Joint Commission, 100-101, 115-117,

at Lutheran General Hospital, 48-54

and organization framework, 69, 75, 93, 101, 118, 128

role of, 6, 7, 68-69, 75, 94, 95, 96, 101

self-assessment of, 102, 112-115t

training of, 95-98, 100, 101, 102

example programs, 96-97, 97t, 98, 99t, 100, 100t

Ethics mechanisms. *See also* Education; Ethics, consultation; Ethics committee; Mission statements; Vision statements designing, 73, 74t, 75, 93, 100-102, 103t, 104-108

educating about, 75-76

evaluating, 84, 102-103, 112-115

implementing, 75, 93-94, 100-102, 104f, 105f, 106-108f, 118

in Joint Commission survey process, 103, 108, 111, 115-117

in organizations, 68, 69, 72, 73, 75-76, 111, 128

Ethics Outreach Services, 98, 99t

Experiments. *See* Research studies

Extraordinary care, versus ordinary, 4

F

Feminist ethics. *See* Ethics of caring

Fidelity, 11-12, 13, 16

Futile treatment, 7-9, 10, 13, 15-16, 36, 126-127

case study about potential for, 7-9, 15-16

G

Geriatrics, 12, 48, 98, 100, 122-123

Good, 5-6, 9-10, 11, 73

common, 6, 10, 36, 121

greatest, 9-10

Grievances, 93, 111, 116, 117. *See also* Conflicts

policy for, 73, 108

resolution of, 23, 28f

H

Hastings Center, The, 6, 94, 96

Health care surrogate, 23, 38f, 49f, 50f, 51f, 52f

Health care treatment directives. *See* Advance directives

Honesty, 12, 70, 73, 76, 80-81f

Hospice care, 4, 8, 48, 77, 79. *See also* Palliative care

case study of potential candidate for, 125-126

components of compliance, 87, 88-89f

and ethics committee training, 98, 99t

example code of ethics, 77, 80-82f

example mission and vision statement for, 75, 77f

and insurance coverage, 31, 35, 125-126

Medicare benefit for, 31, 35

and patient rights, 23, 36

and Patient Self-Determination Act of 1990, 29

Human Genome Project, 96

Human resource management, 68, 73, 74t, 76, 76f, 88-89f

I

Individual good, versus common, 6, 10, 36

Informed consent, 4, 5, 23, 24f, 26f, 31, 38-39f, 102, 110f, 127

and Joint Commission requirements, 21, 108, 117

Informed decision making, sample policy for, 30-31

Institutional Review Board (IRB), 4, 74t

Insurance, 67, 70

and continuing futile care, 126-127

limiting services according to, 125-126

Integrated Ethics program, 96-97

Internet ethics resources, 133

Interviews, in Joint Commission survey process, 115-117

J

Joint Commission on Accreditation of Healthcare Organizations, 23, 69

document review, 108, 111, 115, 117

interviews, in survey process, 115-117

standards of, 3, 13, 21-22, 22t, 72-73, 100-101, 103

survey process of, 103, 108, 111, 115-117

Journals, on patient rights and ethics, 131

K

Kant, Immanuel, 3, 10-11, 17

L

Leadership

and conflicts of interest, 77, 79, 82-83, 83t

ethics education for, 68, 76, 93, 103

and Joint Commission survey process, 103, 108, 111, 115-117

moral, 67, 68, 73

resources for, 42f, 68, 95, 131-135

role of, 7, 54, 67, 75, 86, 87, 95, 118

Legalism. See Positivism

Life-prolonging procedures, 8, 9, 11, 50f, 58f, 126-127

refusing, 45f, 49f, 50-51f

sample policy for, 57f, 94

withholding or withdrawing, 48, 49-52f

Life-sustaining care

refusing, 13, 23, 28f

withholding or withdrawing, 29, 35, 36, 38, 49f, 58f, 108

Living wills, 35, 37f, 43f, 49f, 51f, 56-57f, 63f

incapacitated or incompetent patients with, 51-52f

Long term care facilities. See Nursing homes

M

Marketing, ethics in, 67, 68, 73, 74t, 77, 78-79f, 108, 116, 118

Medicaid, 5, 37-38f

Medical ethics. See Bioethics

Medicare, 5, 29, 31, 35, 37-38f

Midwest Bioethics Center, 23, 26-28f, 29, 30-31f, 32-35f, 36, 37-42f, 43-44f, 45-46f, 102, 112-115f

Minors

decision making guidelines for, 32-35f

parents refusing treatment for, on religious grounds, 127-128

rights of, 29, 32-35f, 38

Misconduct. See Conduct, violations of

Mission statements, 68, 72, 73, 74f, 76, 93, 118

conflict with, 67

developing and implementing, 72, 75

educating staff about, 75-76

examples of, 76f, 77f

in meeting Joint Commission standards, 72, 111

Model for ethical inquiries, 14-17, 121, 122, 128

Moral norms, 12-13

N

Narrative ethics, 6, 14, 17, 121

National Association of Home Care, 23

National Association of Social Workers, 29

National Commission for the Protection of Human Subjects of Biomedical and Behavioral Research, 4

National Hospice Organization, 23, 72

Newsletters, on patient rights
    and ethics, 131

Nonconsequentialism, 10-12, 13

Nonmaleficence, 6, 11, 12, 16, 121

Nuremberg Code, 4

Nursing homes, 3, 29, 39f, 60,
    61f, 77 122-123

    and Medicare funding, 29

    rights of residents, 6, 12, 23, 96

    staff education needs, 96, 98, 100

    and withholding or withdrawing
        life-sustaining care, 48

O

Ordinary care, versus extraordinary, 4

Organ procurement, 4, 22t,
    46f, 100, 108, 117, 126-127

Organ transplantation, 4, 11, 22t

Organization ethics, 7, 67-90

    addressing, 73, 75-76, 100-102

    assessment of, 94-95, 102-103

    case study on, 124-125

    considerations for, 69-70, 71t,
        74t, 103t

    creating climate for, 7, 67-70, 76-77,
        79, 82-84, 86=87

    educating staff about, 7, 76, 83-84,
        93, 95-98, 100

    and ethics committee, 69, 100-102

    framework for, 73, 75-76, 93-94

    integrating, with clinical ethics,
        67, 69-70, 95

    and Joint Commission, 72-73,
        100, 103, 108, 111, 115-117

    leaders' commitment to, 69, 87

    monitoring performance of, 83-84,
        85f, 86-87, 88-89f, 90f

    statement of, 77, 78-79f, 80-82f, 86f

P

Palliative care, 8, 15, 31, 58f.
    See also Hospice care

    appropriate use of, 29, 35, 48

    case study of, 48, 53-54f, 54,
        55f, 56f, 57f, 125-126

    sample policy for, 53-54f

    standing orders for, 55f

Pamphlets, on patient rights
    and ethics, 62-64f, 131-133

Patient. *See also* Patient rights

    autonomy of, 7, 8, 12, 16, 21, 36,
        84, 100

    in behavioral health care
        organizations, 29, 79, 93

    bill of rights, 22t, 23, 24-25f, 72

    capacity of, 3, 12, 15, 29, 32-35f, 37f, 38f,
        43f, 45f, 50-52f, 108, 110f

    handouts for, 23

    interviews, with Joint
        Commission surveyors, 117

    minors as, 32-35, 38, 127-128

    in nursing homes, 6, 23

    organization obligations to, 7, 93

    relationships with staff, 13, 76, 77,
        79, 82, 95, 96, 100

    responsibilities, 3, 6, 23, 25f, 27-28f,
        29, 60, 62-63f, 117

        documents on, 21, 22t, 23, 108, 117

    terminally ill, 4, 6, 11, 31, 45f, 54,
        56-59f, 121

Patient rights, 12, 13, 21, 36,
    62-63f, 100t

    addressing, 21, 93, 100-102, 116, 117

    and advance directives, 24f, 27f,
        35-36, 37-41f, 49f, 94, 116, 117

    and American law, 4

    applying to clinical policies and
        procedures, 21-64

bill of, 22t
of American Hospital Association, 23, 24-25f, 72
of National Association of Home Care, 23
documents, 22t, 23, 24-25f, 29, 60, 93, 108, 118, 128
educating patients to, 23, 111, 117
educating staff to, 93, 95-98, 100, 111
and Joint Commission standards, 3, 21, 72, 73, 100, 103, 108, 111, 115-117
of minors, 29, 32-35f
movement, 3-5
policies, 5, 26-28f, 60, 115
respect for, 13, 21, 22, 84
sample brochure, 62-64f
statements, 23
Patient Self-Determination Act (PSDA) of 1990, 4, 27f, 29, 35, 37-42f, 59, 94
Philosophy
and bioethics, 3-4, 5, 10, 22, 93, 96
of hospice, 23, 126
organization, 21
personal, 9, 14, 16, 95
Philosophy statements, 3, 4, 48, 60, 68, 75, 76f, 95, 115.
Physicians. See also Staff
autonomy of, 8, 16, 36
and beneficence, 7, 8, 11, 16, 121
communications with patients, 8, 12, 13, 15, 16, 29, 31, 125-126
conflicts of interest, 82, 83, 84t, 95
and financial partnerships, 67, 87
and Medicare, 5, 31
obligations of, 8, 12, 13, 16, 36, 70, 127-128
Positivism, 12-13, 17

Power of attorney. See Durable power of attorney for health care
President's Commission on the Study of Ethical Problems in Medicine and Biomedical and Behavioral Research, 4
Privacy, 4, 12, 21, 23, 24f, 26f, 34f, 62f, 100t, 117, 123
Professional codes. See Code of ethics, professional
Professional societies and associations, 23, 29, 36, 48, 72, 96, 135
Proxy, 49f, 50f, 51f, 52f, 57f
Public relations, 79t, 93

Q
Quality of life, 6, 8, 126
Quinlan, Karen Ann, 4, 29, 113f

R
Records
accuracy of, 70, 71t
audits of, 54, 56-59f
Refusal of treatment, 13, 34f, 35, 45f, 49f, 50-51f, 122-123, 127-128
consequences of, 23, 28f
with medications, 6, 29
Religion, role in ethics, 3-4, 8, 15, 23, 75, 93, 96, 97, 100, 116, 126-128
Reproductive technology, 100
Research studies, patient participation in, 4, 13, 25f, 29, 31, 32f, 34f, 62f, 100t, 108
Resident. See Patient
Resources
allocation of, 4, 5, 8, 16, 70, 72, 81-82f, 84
educational, 93, 95-98
health care, limited, 10, 70, 126-127
on patient rights and ethics, 129-135
Resuscitation policies, 5, 16, 36, 108. See also Do-not-resuscitate orders

Rights documents. *See* Patient rights, documents

S

Self-determination, 4, 5, 8, 11, 12-13, 16, 36, 43f, 48

Staff, 6, 67, 69, 75, 76, 77, 87, 93-94,
    competence, 70
    conflicts of interest, 7, 68, 73, 77, 79, 82-83, 83t, 84t, 111
    education of, 21, 41f, 54, 59, 60, 68, 76, 83-84, 93, 94-98, 100-102, 111, 113-114f, 117, 118, 121
    interviews with Joint Commission surveyors, 21, 115-117
    relationships, with patients, 76, 77, 79
    responsibilities, 67, 70, 82, 195
    rights of, 80f, 84, 93

Stewardship, 7, 70, 73, 75, 76-77, 78f,

Study to Understand Prognoses and Preferences for Outcomes and Risks of Treatment (SUPPORT), 29, 31, 48

T

Teleological ethics. *See* Consequentialism

Terminal illness
    in advance directives, 45f
    and hospice care, 4, 6, 31
    and palliative care, 54, 56-59f
    and requests for cardiopulmonary resuscitation, 8, 11, 121

Third-party payers. *See* Insurance

Training. *See* Education

Treatment directives. *See* Advance directives

U

Universality, 11

Utilitarianism, 9, 13

V

Values, 3, 5, 6, 10-11, 36, 67, 72, 75, 77
    analysis of, 7-9, 14-17, 75, 94-95, 121-128
    of health care workers, 16, 83, 93, 94, 97, 103
    of organizations, 68, 72, 73, 75, 76
    of patients, 8, 14, 67
    training, 83-84, 85f, 86-87, 95-98, 98t, 99t

Values statements, 7, 68, 69, 72, 73, 74t, 76, 93, 111, 118.
    clarifying, 75-76, 78-79f
    developing, 75
    examples of, 77f, 80-82f, 106f

Vision statements, 13, 72, 74t, 75.
    examples of, 77, 80f

W

Withdrawing or withholding treatment or care, 5, 35, 36, 45f, 48, 54, 55f, 108
    in advance directives, 45f
    in case study, 16, 125-126, 126-127
    and legal cases, 29
    position statements on, 48
    sample policy, 48, 49-52f

Woodstock Theological Center, 69-70, 71t